A STUDENT'S GUIDE TO EXERCISE FOR IMPROVING HEALTH

**Matthew D. McCabe, Ph.D. and
Bradley R. A. Wilson, Ph.D.**

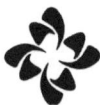

❖ cognella® | ACADEMIC PUBLISHING

Bassim Hamadeh, CEO and Publisher
Kassie Graves, Acquisitions Editor
Berenice Quirino, Associate Production Editor
Miguel Macias, Senior Graphic Designer
Alexa Lucido, Licensing Associate
Don Kesner, Interior Designer
Natalie Piccotti, Senior Marketing Manager
Kassie Graves, Director of Acquisitions and Sales
Jamie Giganti, Senior Managing Editor

Cover image copyright© 2017 iStockphoto LP/Cecilie_Arcurs.

Printed in the United States of America

ISBN: 978-1-5165-2438-9 (pbk)

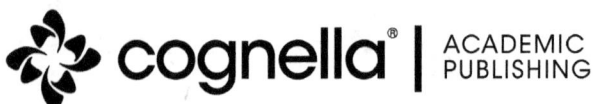

cognella® | ACADEMIC PUBLISHING

A STUDENT'S GUIDE TO EXERCISE FOR IMPROVING HEALTH

DEDICATION

Dedicated to Forrest, Anita, and Mark McCabe and Andrea Nicholson for their continuous love and support. MM

Dedicated to Gene and Darlene Wilson for their unending love, guidance, and support. BW

THE COGNELLA SERIES ON STUDENT SUCCESS

S tudent success isn't always measured in straight As.

Many students arrive at college believing that if they study hard and earn top grades, their higher education experience will be a success. Few recognize that some of their greatest learning opportunities will take place outside the classroom. Learning how to manage stress, navigate new relationships, or put together a budget can be just as important as acing a pop quiz.

The Cognella Series on Student Success is a collection of books designed to help students develop the essential life and learning skills needed to support a happy, healthy, and productive higher education experience. Featuring topics suggested by students and books written by experts, the series offers research-based, yet practical advice to help any student navigate new challenges and succeed throughout their college experience.

Series Editor: Richard Parsons, Ph.D.
Professor of Counselor Education, West Chester University

Other titles available in the series:

- *A Student's Guide to Stress Management*
- *A Student's Guide to a Meaningful Career*
- *A Student's Guide to College Transition*
- *A Student's Guide to Self-Care*
- *A Student's Guide to Money Matters*
- *A Student's Guide to Communication and Self-Presentation*

ABOUT THE AUTHORS

Most college students know that regular exercise can improve their health and overall well-being, but with essays to write, labs to complete, and chapters to read before class, who has time to exercise? You do!

A Student's Guide to Exercise for Improving Health provides you with practical advice and suggestions that will help you balance a healthy, active lifestyle with academic success. You'll learn about a myriad benefits of exercise on your mental, emotional, and physical well-being, how to design an exercise program that works with your course schedule, and how to set realistic and attainable fitness goals that will improve your health and happiness.

In helping you to develop healthy habits and a regular exercise program, this guide will help you achieve goals related not only to physical fitness, but to academic success as well.

A Student's Guide to Exercise for Improving Health is part of the Cognella Series on Student Success, a collection of books designed to help students develop the essential life and learning skills needed to support a happy, healthy, and productive higher education experience.

Matthew D. McCabe is a visiting professor of exercise science at Tiffin University. He earned his bachelor's degree in sports management with a concentration in exercise science from Wilmington College, his master's degree in clinical exercise physiology from Ohio University, and his doctoral degree in health education from the University of Cincinnati.

Bradley R. A. Wilson is a professor of health promotion and education at the University of Cincinnati. He earned his master's in business administration and his Ph.D. in exercise science from Michigan State University. Dr. Wilson has authored or co-authored over 60 papers and book chapters on health care in the U.S., kinesiology, the health and fitness industry, healthy lifestyles, performance-enhancing drugs, and more. He has presented on health and exercise topics throughout the U.S., Europe, South America, and Asia.

CONTENTS

EDITOR'S PREFACE

The transition to college marks a significant milestone in a person's life. Many of you will be preparing to live away from your friends and family for the very first time. Clearly this is and should be an exciting time.

It is a time to experience new things and experiment with new options. While the opportunity to grow is clear—so too are the many challenges you will experience as you transition from high school to college.

Research suggests that the first year of college is the most difficult period of adjustment a student faces. Not only will you be required to adjust to new academic demands but you will also have to navigate a number of social and emotional challenges that accompany your life as a college student. The books found within this series—*Congella Series on Student Success*—have been developed to help you with the many issues confronting your successful transition from life as a high school student to life as a collegiate. Each book within the series was designed to provide research-based, yet *practical* advice to assist you succeeding in your college experience.

As you transition to college it will become clear that there is much to do and often little time to do it. Given all that is currently on your things to do list, as well as the many more things to be added once you set foot on campus, you may find that exercising has fallen to the bottom of the list, if it ever was on the list. The research is abundant in regard to the downside to a sedentary lifestyle. Yet even with the wealth of information pointing to the benefits of exercise to one's health and well-being, the data continues to show that many young people fail to meet the minimum exercise recommendations established by the American Heart Association and the American College of Sports Medicine. Yes there is much to do—but caring for your health is essential to the completion of all the other things on your "to do list" and exercise is a valuable resource for taking care of your health.

The current book, *A Student's Guide to Exercise for Improving Health*, provides you with well-researched, practical advice for developing and maintaining a healthy lifestyle through exercise. As you will soon come to discover, while the topic is serious, the manner in which the information is presented is both engaging and directly applicable to your own current life experience. The book employs case illustrations in a feature called *"Voices From Campus"* and opportunities to apply what you are learning in a feature called *"Your Turn."*

I know that you will find this, as well as the other books within the series, to be a useful guide to your successful transition from high school to college.

Richard Parsons, Ph.D.
Series Editor

AUTHORS' PREFACE

E xercise is a subject that many people know something about but in many ways is misunderstood. We are constantly bombarded with information about how to best exercise and which programs work the best, but it is difficult to know which information to believe. The global health and fitness club industry has revenues over $80 billion and that does not include equipment, clothing, videos, software, and other related products. With so much opportunity to make money there are many products and services that make false claims.

While exercise has many health benefits, if done improperly injuries and health complications can occur. While this is a reason some do not exercise, it should not be an excuse. Almost everyone can do some form of exercise safely!

The reason we wrote this book is to help young people get started in and maintain an effective exercise program. Getting a personal trainer to assess your fitness level and help you develop your exercise program is beneficial but costly. For most healthy people that would be convenient and useful but it is not necessary. With a little understanding of exercise and good planning practices you can develop your own healthy exercise program. Just follow the steps outlined in this book. Although exercise is scientific, the information is presented in basic terms. The assessments are simple and can be done at home. Appropriate goals can be determined and the proper exercise program can be designed. The various types of exercises and classes are also presented to help find activities that are fun and motivating. However, describing each type of resistance and flexibility exercise available goes beyond the scope of this book. To help find specific exercises, keywords to search the Internet are provided.

Throughout the book you will find information to support your learning and exercise program development. *"Myth Boxes"* will help to clarify some of the major misunderstandings about exercise and fitness. Exercise experiences will be told in *"Voices From Campus."* Additionally, there are *"Supplement Your Learning"* sections for added detail and understanding. But the most important exercises are *"Your Turn"* where you have the opportunity to apply what you learned to the development of your own personalized exercise program.

The health benefits of exercise can be obtained by virtually everyone. The most important factor is to develop your program and get started. The result will most certainly be a healthier life. Happy exercising!

INTRODUCTION TO EXERCISE AND HEALTH

I am already healthy so why do I need to exercise?

Very strong evidence suggests that regular participation in planned exercise and engaging in physical activity are associated with a myriad of positive health-related outcomes. These health-related benefits include, but are not limited to, reduction in the risk for developing cardiovascular disease, type 2 diabetes mellitus, colon and breast cancer, obesity and overweightness, depression and anxiety, and all-cause and premature death. Moreover, there is strong-to-moderate evidence that with increasing levels of exercise, physical activity, and fitness the achievement of the previously mentioned health-related benefits are more pronounced.

However, despite the known health-related benefits, exercise participation and physical activity rates in the United States are alarmingly low. According to the Centers for Disease Control and Prevention nearly 80 percent of adults 18 years and older fail to meet the minimum exercise recommendations established by the American Heart Association and the American College of Sports Medicine.[2] These recommendations state that healthy adults should participate in moderately intense aerobic exercise for at least 150 minutes per week with an additional program of resistance exercises two or three days per week.[3] Additionally, approximately 24 percent of all adults in the United States are completely inactive.[2] In short, research shows that more adults in the United States are completely inactive than those who meet the minimum exercise dose for achieving optimal health-related benefits. The public health consequences for a "lack" of physical activity are clear. Physical inactivity feeds into obesity which feeds into high blood fat levels (dyslipidemia) which feeds into high blood pressure and high blood sugar (glucose) which ultimately feeds cardiovascular diseases. So physical inactivity is a major contributor to obesity which provides fuel to the fires of disease, particularly cardio-metabolic diseases (mentioned above) as it helps drive the heart disease process. Simply by moving more and being more physically active as a society, 6 to 10 percent of the worldwide cases of coronary artery disease, type 2 diabetes, colon and breast cancer, and premature mortality could be eliminated.

Transitioning to college includes many lifestyle changes. Food is readily available in the residence halls, including unhealthy food choices. Many students who played high school sports are no longer getting regular, organized physical activity. Time spent in classrooms decreases but time needed to study increases. With change comes some stress. Students who eat more calories and spend less time exercising will gain weight. The average 15 pounds of weight gain during the freshman year is often called the "Freshman 15!"

Establishing positive exercise behaviors at a younger age is very important. When examining the college population, nearly half of all college students fail to meet the minimum exercise recommendations listed above.[4] This is certainly a higher level of exercise participation than in the general adult population; however, for the near 50 percent of college students not meeting the minimum exercise recommendations there is a long-term health risk. According to research this risk exists because there is an inverse relationship between physical activity and age. Simply put, on average, as college students graduate and progress in age they are more likely to exercise less than in the past. This is a health risk because decreases in physical activity are correlated to the development of numerous chronic diseases. Therefore, it is critical that college students equip themselves with the knowledge and skills needed to initiate and execute their own exercise plan with the goal of improving or sustaining health. After graduation it is easier to sustain good habits developed in college than change bad habits!

1.1: Physical Activity and Exercise

When communicating with patients, clients, and the population, exercise professionals often use the terms physical activity and exercise interchangeably. However, there are distinct differences between physical activity and exercise. Physical activity refers to bodily movements produced by muscular contractions which elevate metabolic demands such as heart rate, respiration, or caloric expenditure. Examples of physical activity include playing a round of golf, a pickup game of basketball, or even strenuous manual labor. Exercise, on the other hand, refers to a specific form of physical activity in which movements are planned, structured, and repetitive with the goal of improving or maintaining one or more components of physical fitness. Therefore, the distinction between physical activity and exercise is intent. Do people intend to complete physical activity for fun or leisure? Or do they intend to engage in planned and rigidly structured forms of physical activity as a means of improving their health?

While physical activity, in general, can improve health, there needs to be a conscious effort to modulate the frequency, time, and intensity of physical activity. Research indicates a dose-response relationship between the amounts of physical activity people get and the benefits achieved. That is, the more physical activity people get, the lower their risk for developing a laundry list of preventable diseases, mainly cardiovascular disease. Further, it is important to modulate the frequency, time, and intensity of physical activity because it is the level of physical fitness, and not necessarily the cumulative amount of physical activity, that has the greater impact on health. Therefore, future chapters in this text will provide techniques for implementing physical activity and exercise plans in which components of physical fitness can be optimally improved and thereby influence long-term health.

College Students Exercising

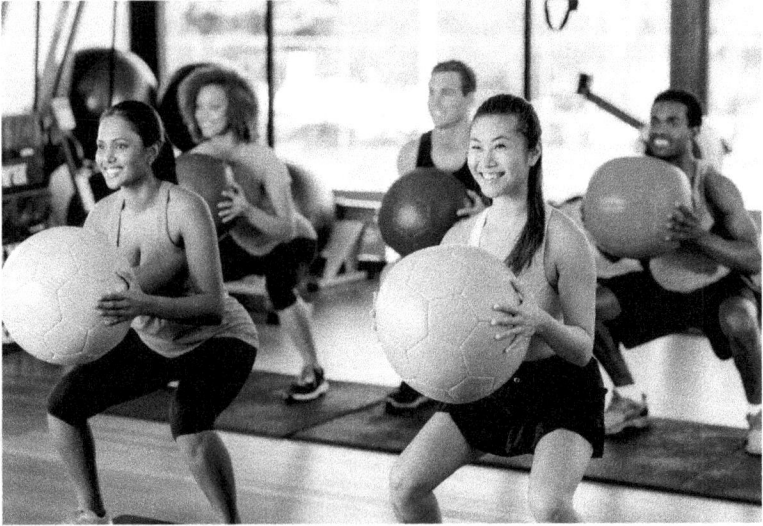

Students Playing Pick-up Basketball

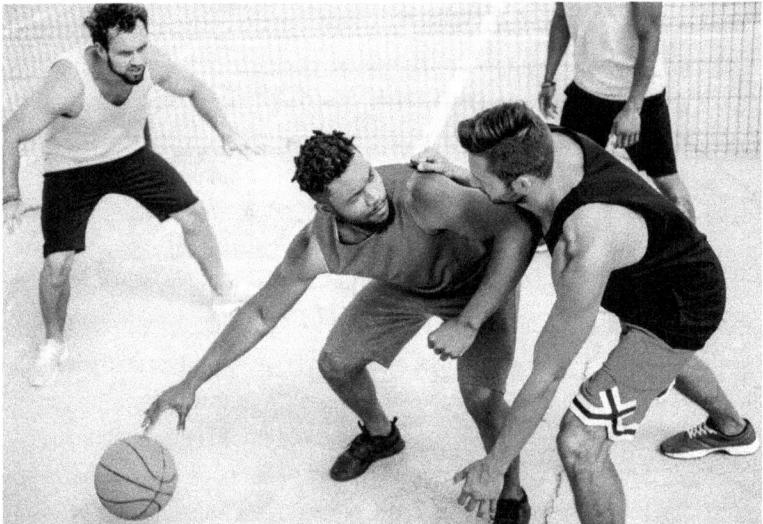

YOUR TURN 1.1

Exercise and Physical Activity

Directions: The terms "exercise" and "physical activity" have been defined. Think of different activities that would fall into each of these categories. First, put each activity below into the correct category. Then in each category add two activities that are not included on the list.

Categorize the following:
Seven stretches
Tennis
Yoga
Mowing the lawn
Downhill skiing
Nine resistance training lifts
Walking up the stairs to class
Riding a stationary bicycle

Exercise	Physical Activity
1.	1.
2.	2.
3.	3.
4.	4.
5.	5.
6.	6.
7.	7.
8.	8.

1.2: Effects of Exercise on Health

There are countless health-related benefits that can be achieved through participation in a well-designed exercise program. Most college students are likely familiar with the facts that exercise improves cardiovascular health and can aid in the loss or maintenance of body fat. However, exercise affects far more aspects of health. Regular exercise can influence mood, brain performance, and joint health. These are just a few of the wide-reaching health-related benefits associated with exercise. The following section discusses how regular exercise can influence several aspects of health.

Exercise and Cardiovascular Disease

Cardiovascular disease is a far-reaching term which describes any disease affecting the heart and blood vessels. When cardiovascular diseases are combined together they make up the leading cause of death in the United States, slightly ahead of cancer. Common cardiovascular diseases include coronary artery disease (blocked arteries which deliver blood to the heart muscle), cerebrovascular disease (blocked arteries which deliver blood to the brain), peripheral artery disease (blocked arteries which deliver blood to the skeletal muscles), and hypertension (high blood pressure). At the center of many cardiovascular diseases is atherosclerosis. Atherosclerosis is a condition in which fatty deposits form in blood vessels and disrupt the flow of blood. These atherosclerotic plaque deposits can build up to the point that they block (occlude) blood flow or the deposits can aid in blood clot formation leading to a blockage at that site or somewhere "downstream" in the blood vessels. While healthy lifestyle choices such as eating a low-fat diet rich in fruits and vegetables and abstaining from tobacco use are helpful in preventing cardiovascular disease, a lack of physical activity and low levels of physical fitness are the most powerful predictors for developing cardiovascular disease. In fact, someone who is lean and eats a healthy diet but who does not get enough physical activity and has a low level of fitness is at greater risk of premature mortality from cardiovascular disease than someone who smokes and eats a bad diet but gets a lot of physical activity and has a high level of fitness. Furthermore, it is estimated that if every adult in the United States adhered to the minimum exercise recommendations of getting at least 150 minutes of moderately intense aerobic exercise per week, nearly 30 percent of deaths from coronary artery disease and nearly 25 percent of deaths from stroke would be prevented.[6] These findings underscore the importance of regular exercise as a means of preventing cardiovascular disease.

A heart attack is the result of severe cardiovascular disease. But it is important to realize that although a heart attack happens suddenly, it has actually been progressing silently for decades. Most college-aged students have some plaque deposits which currently cause no health complications. But in the future they will continue to accumulate plaque which eventually could lead to a heart attack. Therefore, starting an exercise program while in college can slow the progression of cardiovascular diseases while also developing positive exercise habits to maintain good health in the future!

Before explaining how exercise reduces the risk of cardiovascular disease it is useful to have a working knowledge of the cardiovascular system. The primary purpose of the cardiovascular system is to supply oxygen and nutrient-rich blood to the cells in the body. At the center of the cardiovascular system, the heart acts as the pump that pushes blood first to the lungs in order to pick up oxygen and then to the rest of the body where that oxygen is used to construct small molecules needed to fuel bodily functions. The cardiovascular system also contains arteries and veins. The arteries deliver oxygen and nutrient-rich blood to working tissues and the veins transport blood back to the heart. Virtually all cells in the human body require oxygen to survive and function; thus a healthy cardiovascular system, consisting of a strong efficient heart and clear and compliant (flexible) blood vessels, is essential for sustaining life.

The heart is a muscle that contains four chambers and works non-stop. It contracts between 60 and 100 times per minute, every minute of every day. That is over 35 million times per year! With all of this work, the heart requires a steady supply of oxygen and nutrients, such as fats and carbohydrates for energy, to continuously support the rest of the body's needs. The heart receives its oxygen and nutrients via the coronary arteries. The coronary arteries are a network of blood vessels that arise from the top of the heart. So the heart pumps its own blood supply! The coronary arteries are the most common site for cardiovascular disease to take place. Here, buildup of atherosclerotic plaque can impede the flow of oxygen-rich blood to specific areas of the heart muscle. This impediment of blood acts to "starve" areas of the heart from oxygen and, as a result, a myocardial infarction (heart attack) can occur. A myocardial infarction is an event in which heart muscle cells die and can no longer contribute to the overall contraction and pumping efforts of the heart. This means the heart will have a limited ability to support the body's oxygen and nutrient needs. If a large enough area of the heart is subjected to prolonged periods of oxygen starvation, then a major heart attack can ensue and lead to death or major disability.

Regular exercise has a major influence on cardiovascular health in a number of ways. As it pertains to the development of coronary artery disease, the most common cardiovascular disease, regular exercise reduces the rate at which atherosclerotic plaque builds up in the coronary arteries. Atherosclerotic plaque is a mixture of fatty materials and white blood cells which hardens and forms occlusions which block blood flow through the blood vessels. Exercise helps reduce atherosclerotic plaque buildup by increasing the breakdown (metabolism) of fats in the blood. When a person exercises, the muscles need energy, and one way the muscles get energy is through breaking down fats. During exercise, fatty acids in triglycerides (fats in the blood) and LDL cholesterol (bad cholesterol) are released and the remnants provide the building blocks for HDL cholesterol (good cholesterol). In essence, regular exercise helps lower the amounts of fat and bad cholesterol in the blood and as a result there is less fat in the blood that can cause atherosclerotic plaque buildup in the coronary arteries.

Atherosclerosis plaque buildup is not exclusive to just the coronary arteries; it can also form in other blood vessels. When atherosclerotic plaque builds up in the carotid arteries (arteries in the neck leading to the brain) or in blood vessels in the brain this condition is called cerebrovascular disease. Cerebrovascular disease, like coronary artery disease, can lead to occlusion of blood vessels and result in oxygen and nutrient starvation. In this case the brain is being deprived. If areas of the brain are deprived of oxygen for too long an ischemic (lack of oxygen) stroke can occur and brain tissue subsequently dies. Regular exercise reduces the risk of cerebrovascular disease in a similar manner to which it reduces the risk of coronary artery disease.

Similar to coronary artery disease and cerebrovascular disease, when atherosclerotic plaque builds up in the arteries of the extremities, mainly the legs, the condition is called peripheral artery disease. Occlusions in the peripheral arteries deprive skeletal muscles and other tissues of the oxygen needed to sustain work. For instance, walking is an activity that is often taken for granted; however, for persons with peripheral artery disease, walking can be an incredibly painful experience. Individuals with peripheral artery disease may only be able to walk for a short distance, at a very slow pace, until the muscles in their legs start to burn and hurt due to a buildup of lactic acid. This pain is similar to the pain in the legs of a healthy person who is sprinting until fatigued. Furthermore, severe peripheral artery disease may result in the need to amputate limbs. Regular exercise reduces the risk of developing peripheral artery disease in the same manner that it reduces the risk for coronary artery disease and cerebrovascular disease.

Hypertension is a condition in which the blood pressure is elevated over a period of time. Blood pressure represents the changing forces of blood against the artery walls as the heart contracts and relaxes. There are two main types of blood pressure: systolic blood pressure (top number) and diastolic blood pressure (bottom number). Systolic blood pressure is representative of the pressure within the aorta (the exiting artery from the heart) during cardiac contraction (systole). Diastolic blood pressure is representative of the pressure within the aorta during the cardiac relaxation (diastole). In general, systolic blood pressure reflects how hard the heart has to work to pump blood throughout the body and diastolic blood pressure is an indicator of the resistance of blood flow through peripheral arteries. While the cause of most cases of hypertension is unknown, elevated blood pressure has a well-documented impact on the development of cardiovascular disease.

High blood pressure plays a critical role in developing atherosclerosis. High blood pressure can damage artery walls thus allowing fats and white blood cells to penetrate the artery walls and begin the process of

Patient Getting Blood Pressure Measured

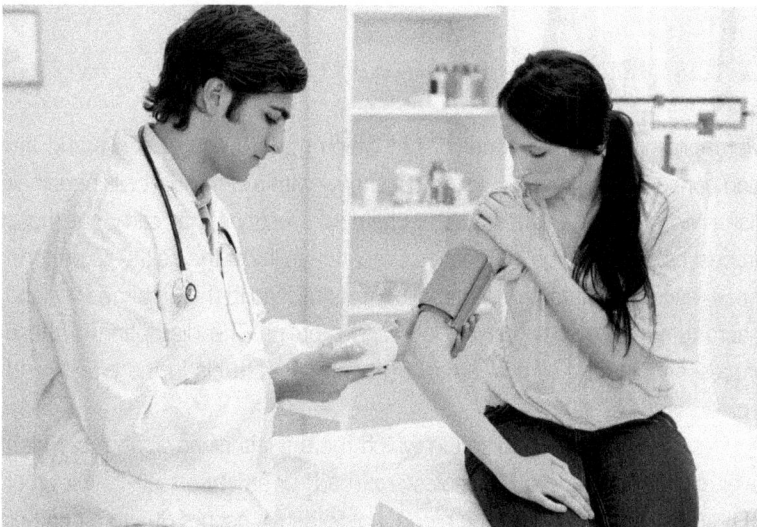

atherosclerotic plaque accumulation. In this regard, regular exercise can help curtail high blood pressure's effect on atherosclerosis by limiting the amounts of fats and bad cholesterol in the blood. High blood pressure also has a negative impact on the heart muscle. The heart muscle, like skeletal muscle, adapts to applied forces. Similar to how skeletal muscle gets bigger in response to resistance training, the heart muscle can enlarge in response to over-exposure to high blood pressure. This enlargement of the heart decreases the heart's ability to pump out a sufficient amount of blood to meet the body's, including the heart's, oxygen and nutrient needs. A single bout of exercise has the capacity to lower blood pressure for 24–48 hours after the exercise session. During exercise, the rate of blood flow is increased in order to supply more blood to working muscles and meet the metabolic needs of the exercise. This enhanced rate of blood flow causes the release of nitric oxide from the blood vessel walls which causes vaso-dilation (opening of arteries) and ultimately acts to lower blood pressure following exercise. Therefore, if a person exercises regularly, the effects of each exercise session will help lower blood pressure and possibly prevent hypertension.

Although college-aged students do not notice any symptoms of the blood vessels beginning to accumulate plaque, the process has begun. This should not cause immediate alarm but instead support the decision to make positive lifestyle changes which include a planned exercise program!

Exercise and Metabolic Diseases

Metabolic diseases are conditions in which the process of converting the food consumed into a useable form of energy within individual cells becomes disrupted. There are thousands of chemical reactions that carry out these processes, and metabolic diseases affect the ability of the cell(s) to perform these reactions. Ultimately, metabolic reactions lead to the breakdown of the macronutrients: carbohydrates, fats, and proteins. The disruption of these processes can lead to dyslipidemia (abnormal fat levels in the blood) and type 2 diabetes.

Dyslipidemia is a condition in which there is either an abnormally high level of triglycerides or LDL cholesterol (bad) or an abnormally low level of HDL cholesterol (good) in the blood. Dyslipidemia occurs due to a number of reasons. Aside from genetics and other existing disorders, poor diet and a lack of physical activity play critical roles in the development of dyslipidemia. Dyslipidemia contributes to the development of atherosclerosis and type 2 diabetes. High levels of triglycerides and LDL cholesterol in the blood increase the likelihood of fat penetrating the artery walls and causing plaque to build up. Likewise, a low level of HDL cholesterol limits the removal of fats in the blood being transported back to the liver. So regular exercise can combat dyslipidemia by reducing fats circulating in the blood. Regular exercise has a small effect on influencing LDL cholesterol; however, it plays a key role in elevating HDL cholesterol which ultimately helps to reduce the risk of plaque buildup in the coronary, cerebral, and peripheral arteries. Aside from dyslipidemia contributing to atherosclerosis, it also contributes to the development of type 2 diabetes. When excess fats are circulating in the blood, they can deposit in and around skeletal muscle which can interfere with the muscle's ability to pull glucose out of the blood. Therefore, exercise's impact on fats in the blood can help reduce the risk of type 2 diabetes.

Insulin is a hormone secreted by the pancreas which helps to remove glucose from the blood. Type 2 diabetes is a disease in which the amount of sugar or glucose in the blood is consistently high. The cause of this elevation is from the inability of the pancreas to produce and secrete sufficient

Patient Having Glucose Screening

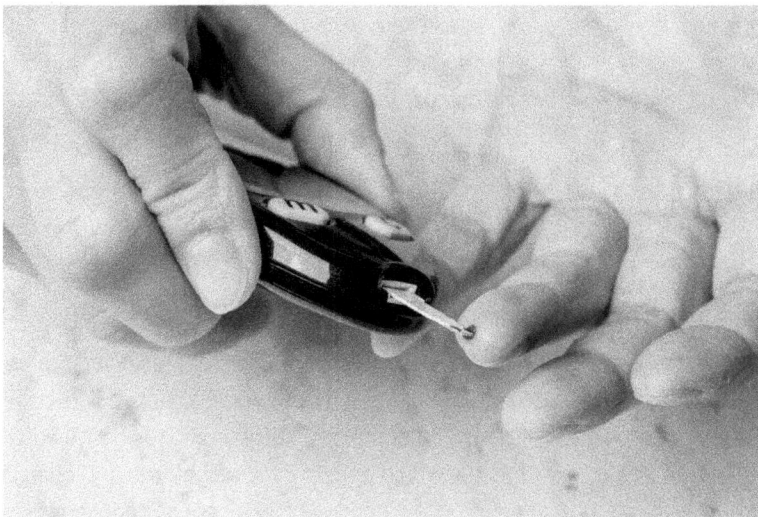

amounts of insulin to help transport the glucose into the cells throughout the body. Type 2 diabetes is a public health crisis as approximately 21 million adults in the United States have a diagnosis of type 2 diabetes, and by the year 2050 it is estimated that 21 percent of the population will have type 2 diabetes.[1, 5] Type 2 diabetes has a profound effect on the development of atherosclerosis as elevated blood glucose can cause vascular damage. Additionally, type 2 diabetes is linked to numerous other diseases such as kidney disease, eye disorders, and various neuropathies (nerve diseases).

Regular exercise has been shown to prevent and slow the progression of type 2 diabetes, reduce medication requirements, and decrease diabetes-related health risks. Additionally, regular exercise has been shown to increase glucose storage in skeletal muscle, glucose transport proteins (proteins that transport glucose across the outer layer of cells), and overall fat metabolism which all act to lower blood glucose levels. What is more important is the muscular contractions involved in exercise allow the uptake of glucose in the muscles without the assistance of insulin! Therefore, consistent participation in exercise and physical activity can help lower blood glucose even if a person has a limited ability to utilize insulin to pull glucose out of the blood, thus highlighting the importance of exercise for the prevention or management of type 2 diabetes.

Like cardiovascular diseases, metabolic diseases take many years of progression to result in disease. Until symptoms of a disease appear it is easy to assume all is well with health. However, the rate of progression is related to many lifestyle choices such as exercise. A regular exercise program can improve the levels of fats and sugars in the blood and slow the progression. Even college-aged students can get these benefits!

Exercise, Fat, and Muscle Mass

In the United States obesity is a major public health issue. Obesity is defined as having a body mass index (height to weight ratio) of 30 kg/m^2 or higher. According to this definition, nearly 37 percent of adults in the United States are classified as obese with an additional 31 percent of adults being classified as overweight. This means that approximately two-thirds of the adult population in the United States would benefit from weight loss. In general, obesity is marked by an abnormally high level of fat mass causing a number of significant health consequences. Some of these consequences include type 2 diabetes, cardiovascular diseases, non-alcoholic fatty liver disease, sleep apnea, colon and breast cancer, orthopedic ailments, increased mortality and morbidity rates, and soaring healthcare costs. Regular exercise is instrumental in preventing fat gain and promoting fat loss. Regular exercise induces fat breakdown and acts to increase the number of destinations for fat breakdown within cells, thereby limiting the amount of fat that gets stored throughout the body.

Not to be overlooked in overall health, the amount of skeletal muscle mass plays an important role in maintaining healthy levels of fat mass, normal levels of fat and glucose in the blood, and sustaining muscular strength. The influence of muscle mass on health can be explained by research suggesting that skeletal muscle accounts for approximately 40 percent of body mass and 30 percent of calories burned at rest. This means that the more muscle mass individuals have the more calories they burn at rest, which is critical for maintaining a healthy body composition. Furthermore, skeletal muscle is the primary location for glucose uptake; therefore, more muscle mass is associated with better blood glucose control. Regular exercise, particularly resistance exercise, increases skeletal muscle mass and muscular strength.

Person Resistance Training to Increase Muscle Mass

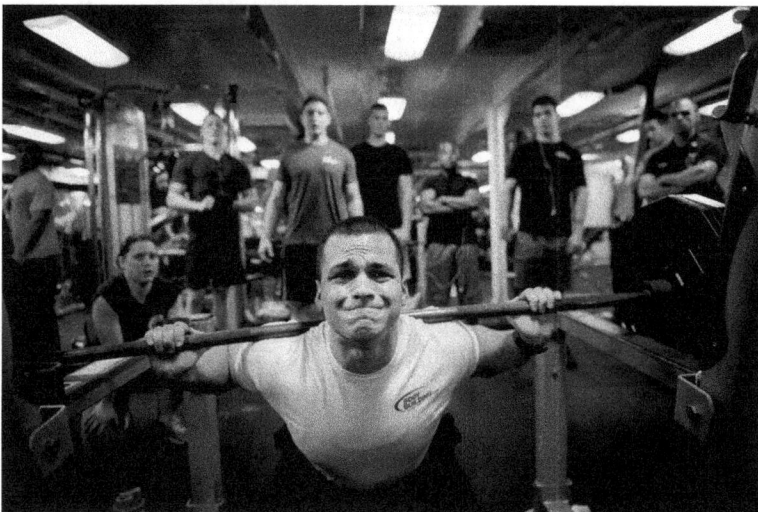

Many college-aged students exercise to improve body appearance. This is a good reason to exercise and it provides motivation. Currently a six-pack above the waist is considered attractive. However, the exercise program should be designed to also improve health. By not following a well-designed program other problems can occur. A hard six-pack may look good but neglect health benefits. Some people go to extremes with exercise by doing too much and can have other more immediate health problems such as too little fat on the body. A well-designed program can include all goals such as health and appearance!

Exercise, Stress, and Mental Health

Mental health can be defined in a number of ways. One way to define mental health is the ability of an individual to cope with issues of everyday life and sustain positive relationships with peers. Disturbances in mental health can be severe enough to warrant a diagnosis of a mental health disorder or may be less severe but nevertheless still have an influence on overall health. Some common disturbances in mental health are stress, anxiety, and depression.

Stress is a part of everyday life and can come in the form of distress (a bad stress) and eustress (a good stress). Examples of common distresses are constantly worrying, anger, or overworking. There is certainly no escape from experiencing distress, but people definitely have control over how often they are exposed to it. Chronic distress can have a negative impact on overall health as it can lead to myocardial infarction, abnormal heart rhythms, and weight gain. From a simplistic standpoint, being in a chronic state of distress causes long-term release of hormones that act to increase blood pressure, accelerate heart rate, and even block fat loss. On the other end of the spectrum, eustress is good and attempts should be made to experience this form of stress as often as possible. The best example of eustress is the stress applied to the body during exercise!

While the research regarding exercise's impact on anxiety and depression is still in its infancy there are plenty of studies that show regular exercise can curtail the sting of anxiety and can help curb symptoms of depression. When a person exercises, the body releases endorphins. Endorphins cause a "feel good" effect, and chronic exposure to these hormones has a positive impact on a person's mood. Additionally, exercise helps the body clear hormones that can have a negative impact on overall health. A very useful benefit of

Students Studying

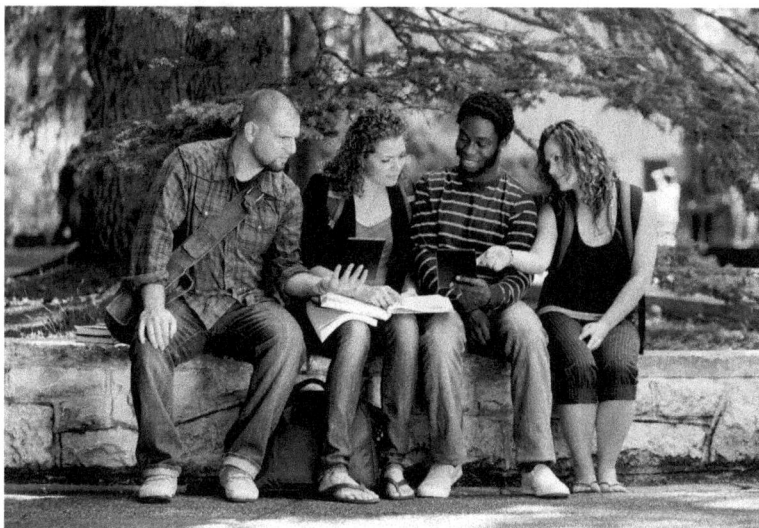

regular exercise for college students, as it pertains to mental health, is that exercise improves the brain's metabolism of glucose which helps improve focus. So before an exam, exercise may help to ace the test! But studying must be done first!

VOICES FROM CAMPUS 1.1

Jackson

I am a freshman in college and starting my second semester. I am a pre-dentistry major and in order for me to get into dental school one day I need to have 3.8 GPA. I did everything I thought I needed to do to get top notch grades. I reviewed my notes, read the books I needed to read, turned in all of my work early, and even studied for tests by writing essays on the topics we were taught. Unfortunately, all this work left me short of my needed 3.8 GPA. While I did have an okay GPA of 3.4, this is still short of my goal.

I talked to my physiology professor about my struggle and he suggested I exercise regularly. "Exercise!" I exclaimed. He said, "Yes, exercise is one of the best things you can do to get that little extra boost on test day." Apparently, exercise helps your brain metabolize glucose and glucose is its preferred fuel.

I trusted my physiology professor and took his advice. I started exercising four days per week and made sure to exercise before taking my exams. Needless to say I started doing better and I am on pace this semester to earn my 3.8 GPA! My advice to other students is be sure to supplement your studying with regular exercise as it can help you stay focused on your studies and on your exams!

Exercise and Cancer

Cancer is a horrific set of diseases that accounts for the second leading cause of death in the United States. It affects nearly everyone in some form or fashion as one in every two men and one in every three women will develop cancer in their lifetime. The pathological process of cancer is very complicated and pinpointing a singular cause is rather difficult. To understand the prevailing theory of how a person develops cancer it is helpful to have an understanding of the cell cycle. The trillions of cells in the human body go through a continuous process of reproduction and programmed death. The reproduction of cells is vital to growth, development, and maintenance of bodily functions (e.g., beating of the heart, breathing, contracting skeletal muscles, etc.). During the cell cycle, cells rely on deoxyribose nucleic acid (DNA) for instructions when dividing. The DNA houses the "blueprint" on how to construct new cells. The prevailing theory of how people develop cancer is that the DNA within cells becomes damaged thus leading to the production of abnormal cells which no longer function as they should. For example a construction worker relies on blueprints for building a bridge. If he or she accidentally spills coffee on the blueprints and tries to construct the bridge from those damaged blueprints, then a mistake may happen resulting in the construction of an unsound bridge. This is essentially what happens to cells when DNA is damaged. The cells will try to repair the damage, but cancer can occur if the cells are unsuccessful. Once cancer begins, the abnormal cells may group together to form a mass known as a tumor, from here further cell division can occur and spread throughout the body.

One way in which cancer is classified is from which type of cell the cancer originates. The most common of these classifications is carcinoma which develops from epithelial cells (the most common type of cell in the human body). Other classifications include leukemia (cancer of blood cells), lymphoma (cancer of immune cells), sarcoma (cancer of connective cells), and melanoma (cancer of skin cells). Further, cancer can impact various anatomical sites such as the lungs, colon, or breasts. Depending on the anatomical location and classification and stage of cancer, survival outcomes can be high or low. For instance carcinoma of the pancreas has one of the lowest five-year survival rates while carcinoma of the prostate gland has one of the highest five-year survival rates. Methods for treating cancer can include surgery, radiation, and chemotherapy. These treatments, in addition to the adverse impacts of the disease, can limit patients' ability to remain physically active.

The effect of exercise on managing cancer is fairly unclear. However, investigations have shown that the better physical fitness people have the better their five-year survival rate. Much of the research regarding exercise and cancer is centered on incident rates and how exercise serves as a

Cancer Survivor who could Benefit from Exercise

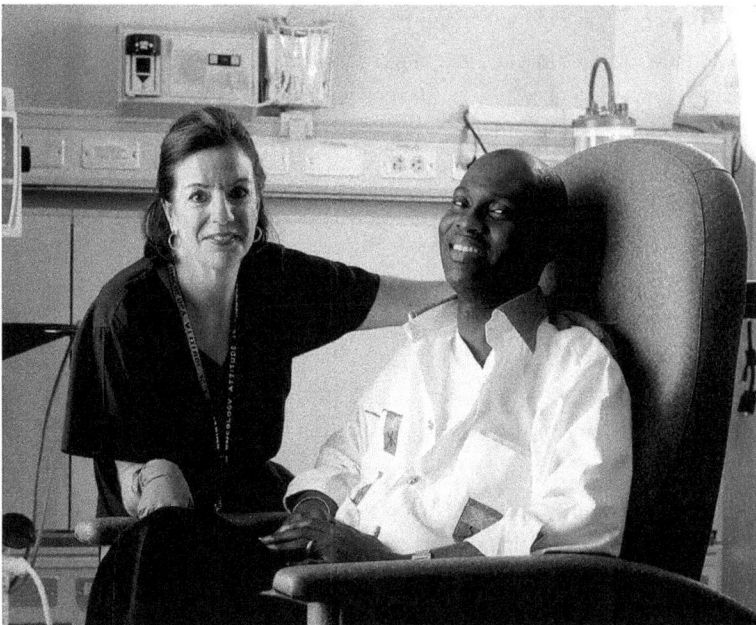

protective mechanism. While regular physical activity has been shown to reduce incident rates of cancer as a whole, it appears to have the strongest preventive influence on colon and breast cancer. There are many proposed mechanisms as to how exercise helps prevent cancer. Some of these mechanisms are improved blood flow and circulation, enhanced immune system capabilities, reduced stress that can damage DNA, and an improved ability of cells to repair damaged DNA. Regardless of the mechanism, the message is fairly clear—exercise can have a profound influence on cancer development. Additionally, those in better health from exercise can tolerate cancer treatments better.

Exercise and Immune Health

One of the most important systems that make up the human body is the immune system. The immune system acts to identify and destroy foreign invaders called pathogens. Pathogens include bacteria, viruses, and fungi and lead to infection if the immune system is unsuccessful in combating their introduction to the body. The most common infection people develop is an upper respiratory tract infection, commonly referred to as the common cold. The common cold is caused by over 200 different viruses. While not usually a danger to survival, the common cold can sideline people from many activities, including exercise. Given that regular exercise is critical to long-term health it is certainly helpful to avoid, as often as possible, developing common infections that can temporarily derail exercise training.

In order to understand how exercise influences the immunity it is useful to have a basic working knowledge of the immune system. The immune system contains both innate (born with it) and adapted or acquired immunity. The innate component of the immune system is composed of physical barriers, specialized cells, and complementary blood-based proteins. These components work in an overlapping fashion to prevent pathogens from invading the body and causing infection. The physical barriers of the immune system consist of the skin and mucous membranes. The skin is the primary barrier along with the mucus that lines our respiratory, urinary, and digestive tracts. Ideally, by maintaining clean and healthy skin, pathogens could be prevented from entering the body. However, some pathogens can enter the body through the mouth, nose, eyes, ears, or the penis or vagina. In this

Person Suffering from a Cold

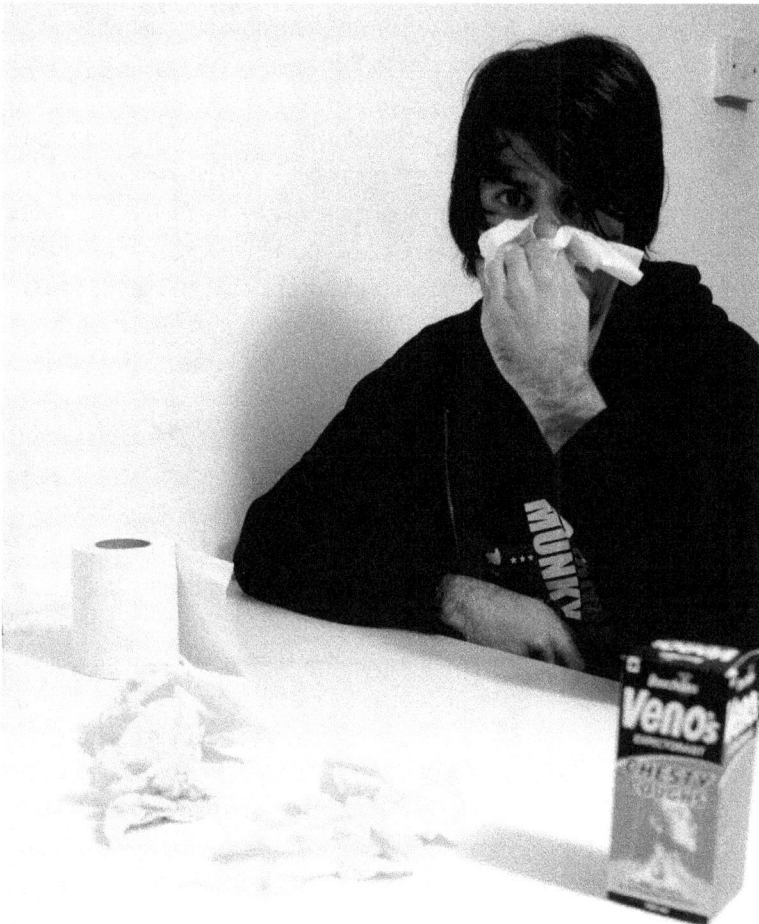

instance, mucous membranes help prevent pathogens from further entry. Beyond these physical barriers there are specialized cells (phagocytes and natural killers) which engulf and destroy pathogens. Third, a series of complementary proteins in the blood circulate and attach themselves to invading pathogens. Here, complementary proteins identify and "tag" foreign invaders so that phagocytes and natural killer cells can find and destroy the pathogens. In addition to the innate immune system, humans also develop immunity to certain pathogens. After exposure to a pathogen, specialized cells act to "remember" the pathogen and develop a stronger defense for the next time the body is exposed to that specific pathogen. This is the process used for vaccinations.

Research indicates that an acute bout of moderately intense aerobic exercise causes an increase in the amount of natural killer cells. However, it appears this elevation in natural killer cells only lasts for a few hours after a single exercise session. Therefore, a single bout of exercise can enhance the defense against pathogens but only temporarily. In addition to aerobic exercise there is evidence to suggest that resistance exercise elicits a similar boost in the immune system, and it too is temporary. In theory, daily physical activity provides people with periods of greater immunity which can reduce the risk for developing common infections such as upper respiratory tract infections. Although exercise can have a direct relationship to enhanced immunity other exercise adaptations like the reduction of stress can play a role in improving the immune system. It is important to complement regular exercise with proper nutrition and sleep to get the most benefit. While exercise does have a positive influence on immunity, exercising too hard and too long negatively affects immunity. Exercise that lasts longer than 90 minutes can decrease the levels of natural killer cells and lead to what is referred to as a window of opportunity for infection. In general, moderately intense exercise lasting between 30 and 60 minutes is very beneficial to immune health.

When people are ill with a cold the question often arises: Should I exercise or not? In general people should never exercise when they have a fever. The best guideline is the above-the-neck rule. If the cold is above the neck in the throat, nose, sinuses, or ears it is generally safe to exercise. Taking it a little easier than normal is fine. Moderate exercise may improve symptoms temporarily. If the cold is below the neck, generally in the lungs, exercise should not be done. It would likely make symptoms worse!

Exercise, Bone, and Joint Health

The human skeletal system has many responsibilities including protecting the internal organs, providing and housing numerous nutrients such as the building blocks for blood cells, and providing the levers needed for

Human Skeleton

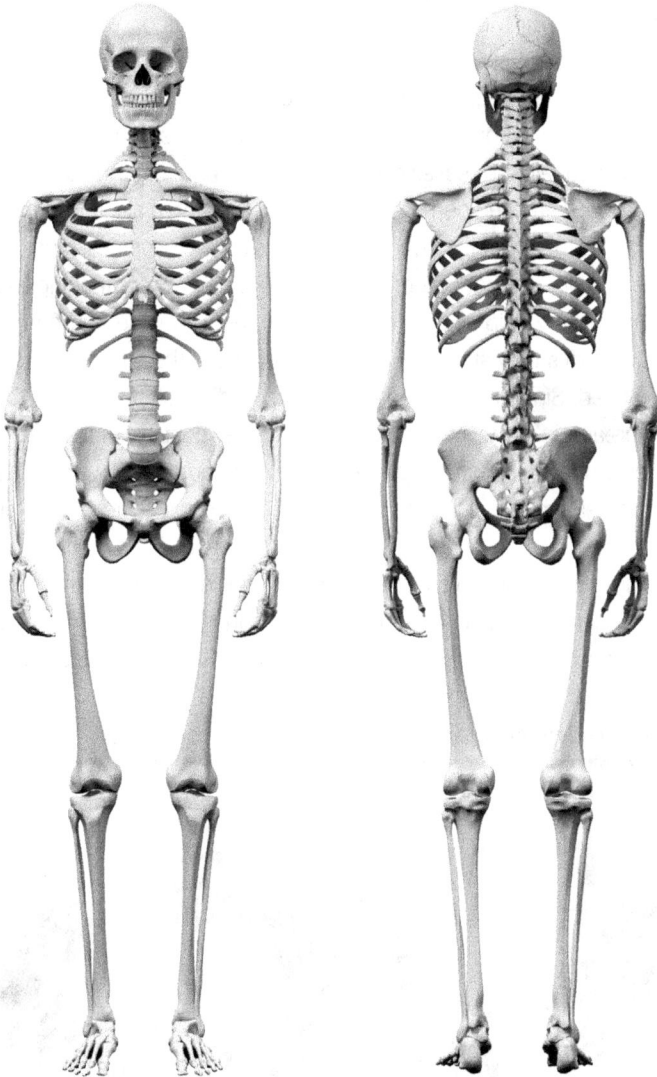

movement. The skeletal system consists of 206 individual bones which combine to form numerous joints and are connected together by ligaments. Maintaining healthy bones and joints is not only crucial for being able to sustain proper movement and functional independence throughout life, but also to continuously replace and replenish blood cells and to promote proper neuromuscular function. A major role of bones is to house calcium which serves a role in repairing and strengthening the bones themselves in addition to providing calcium for nerve conduction and contraction of muscles. Therefore, maintenance or improvements in bone mineral density and the concentration of calcium and other vital minerals within bone are a major necessity for overall health. It is well understood that bone mineral density gradually decreases after the age of 25 and that regular exercise can help minimize these age-related reductions in bone mass and bone mineral density. Further, having strong ligaments helps avoid injuries, long-term joint pain, and joint damage. Exercise plays a key role in strengthening ligaments.

Wolff's Law helps us understand the role of exercise on bone and joint health. Wolff's Law states that bone will adapt to the stresses under which it is placed. Since regular exercise places additional stresses on the bone, an increase in bone mass and bone mineral density can result. Regular exercise that highly stresses the bones and joints (i.e., weight lifting and weight-bearing exercise) can have an osteogenic effect (the formation of new bone tissue). In general, with exercise for improving bone health, specificity, overload, reversibility, and the initial level of bone mass and bone mineral density must be considered. The principles of specificity, overload, and reversibility are discussed later in Chapter 3. For now it is important to

Women Exercising to Improve Bone Mineral Density

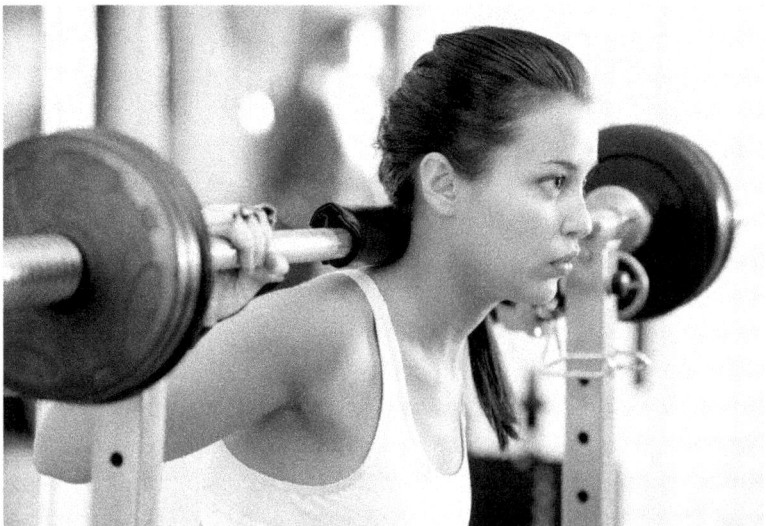

understand that in order for bone to adapt to exercise, the load must be placed on the specific bone to adapt, greater stresses to the bone must be added, when exercise stops the adaptations will be lost, and with lower initial levels of bone mass and bone mineral density prior to training the gains will be greater than when training starts with normal levels of bone mass or bone mineral density.

College-aged students typically have good bone masses. As people age, particularly females, bone mass begins to decrease. If enough bone density is lost, osteoporosis may be diagnosed. Since it is almost impossible to increase bone density in older people, loss of bone mass is permanent. Therefore, college students should exercise regularly to develop good bone mass for later in life! Resistance training exercises are highly recommended.

YOUR TURN 1.2

Identifying How Exercise Can Improve Your Health

Directions: Now that you know the many areas of health exercise can improve, it's time to identify possible areas within your own life that exercise can improve. Please identify five areas of health, in your own life, where exercise can benefit you. An example of this would be a family history of cardiovascular disease. Here, exercise can help reduce your risk for developing the same disease your parents or grandparents have. Also, you may be overweight, suffer from anxiety, or have high blood sugar. Identifying these aspects of your life and health will go a long way when you design your exercise program!

List five areas of health, in your own life, where exercise can benefit you.
1.
2.
3.
4.
5.

Exercise and the Management of Disease

It is well understood that regular exercise has numerous health benefits in addition to serving as a method of disease prevention. However, the general public may be less familiar with the roles exercise can play in the rehabilitation and management of numerous chronic diseases. Exercise is often a part of the treatment strategy for cardiovascular diseases, chronic obstructive pulmonary disease, types 1 and 2 diabetes mellitus, obesity, cancer, multiple sclerosis, Parkinson's disease, fibromyalgia, and osteoarthritis.

Of the many areas of clinical exercise physiology, cardiovascular rehabilitation is arguably the most common. Cardiovascular rehabilitation is an exercise-based rehabilitation program for patients suffering from a myriad of cardiovascular diseases in which exercise is supervised by nurses and clinical exercise physiologists. It is prescribed by a licensed medical physician, oftentimes a cardiologist, for patients with a history of coronary artery disease, myocardial infarction, coronary artery bypass surgery, angioplasty, stable angina (chest pain), peripheral artery disease, heart transplant, stable heart failure, valvular heart surgery, and the implantation of a ventricular assist device (device that helps pump blood). The benefits of cardiovascular rehabilitation are instrumental in achieving positive outcomes following the previously mentioned diagnoses and surgical procedures. These benefits include decreases in angina (chest pain), dyspnea (shortness of breath), fatigue, symptoms of depression, rates of further hospitalization, all-cause mortality, work absence, reoccurrence cardiac events, disease-related progression, and improvements in activities of daily living and the ability of skeletal muscles to use oxygen. As a result of these benefits, many hospitals and medical groups encourage their physicians to consult the cardiovascular rehabilitation team and have them visit patients to educate them on the benefits of cardiovascular rehabilitation. In general, cardiovascular rehabilitation consists of both exercise and educational components and lasts between 12 and 16 weeks.

Another common clinical-based exercise program is pulmonary rehabilitation. Pulmonary rehabilitation, like cardiovascular rehabilitation, is an exercise-based program supervised by nurses and exercise physiologists. Pulmonary rehabilitation is prescribed by licensed physicians, most often for patients diagnosed with chronic obstructive pulmonary disease (COPD).

COPD is a lung disease characterized by the reduction in airflow out of the lungs which results in air being trapped in the lungs, making it challenging to breathe and get oxygen into the blood. Though exercise has little effect on improving COPD, participation in pulmonary rehabilitation helps improve patients' functional fitness, activities of daily living, and the ability of skeletal muscles to utilize oxygen, all of which reduces the stress on the pulmonary system.

Of the many diseases that exercise can help manage, diabetes is one that is potently influenced by regular exercise. While the pathologies of type 1 and type 2 diabetes are very different, they both result in long-term elevations in the concentration of glucose in the blood. Exercise, as discussed earlier in this chapter, elicits glucose uptake into skeletal muscles independent of insulin. The effects of exercise on blood glucose disposal into skeletal muscles can last 24 to 72 hours after a single bout of exercise. Therefore, repeated bouts of exercise can help diabetics maintain normal concentrations of blood glucose.

Other conditions in which physicians may recommend exercise are cancer, multiple sclerosis, Parkinson's disease, fibromyalgia, and osteoarthritis. For cancer, exercise has no known impact on the disease itself, however exercise does increase five-year survival rates, increase quality of life, reduce

Cardiac Rehabilitation Class

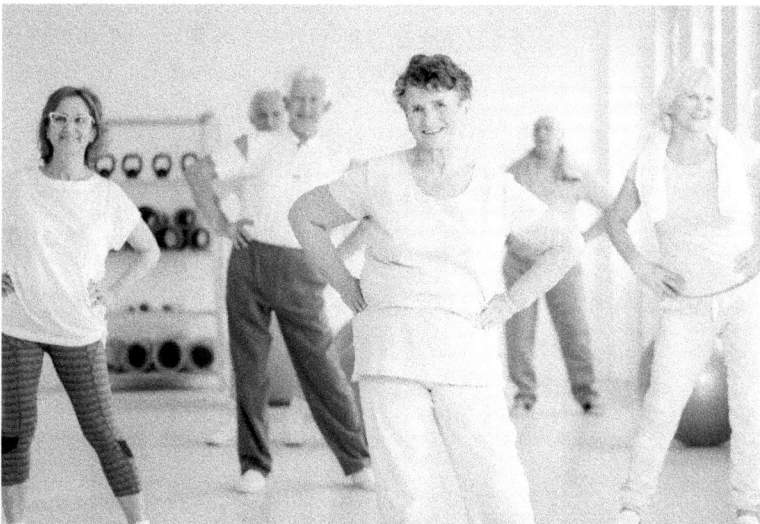

MYTH BOX: NO PAIN, NO GAIN! MORE EXERCISE IS BETTER

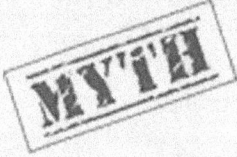

Given the known dose-response relationship between the amount of exercise you get and the benefits you achieve you would think that more exercise is always better and that you could and should always exercise through the pain. However, this notion is entirely false. In fact, exercising more than five days per week offers little to no "extra" health benefit. Consider the law of diminishing returns. This law, in the exercise world, essentially means that at a certain point the benefits of exercise are not increased with continued training. Also, the pain you feel during exercise is a signal that something could be wrong. For instance, pain may mean you have an injury or are experiencing symptoms of something more severe. The wise thing to do when you feel pain during exercise is to slow down or lighten the load. If pain continues, then seek medical consultation.

From an adaptation standpoint, exercise causes the breakdown of muscular proteins, and it is during the synthesis of new proteins where adaptations occur. If you exercise too much, like exercising through pain for instance, the breakdown in proteins could outpace the synthesis of proteins thus leading to a failure to improve—you may even get worse with exercise. As a general rule, exercising three to five days per week is best for health!

disease-related symptoms, and increase exercise tolerance. With multiple sclerosis, an inflammatory disease affecting the nervous system leading to several symptoms including weakness and fatigue, regular exercise has been shown to reduce symptoms of fatigue and improve daily function. Research examining exercise adaptations in Parkinson's disease patients continues to increase. Parkinson's disease is a neurodegenerative disorder which leads to slowed movement and muscle stiffness. Exercise has been shown to improve walking performance, improve quality of life, and reduce the severity of Parkinson's disease. And lastly, with fibromyalgia and osteoarthritis regular exercise is critical in managing pain and progression.

There are many other ailments in which exercise is beneficial. Research will continue to explore exercise as a form of treatment for the diseases discussed in this section and many more. At this point, the message is clear: exercise is a powerful stimulus for promoting positive health-related adaptations and managing several chronic illnesses.

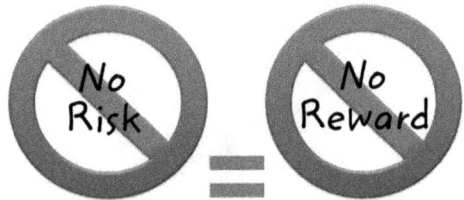

1.3: The Take Away

- Physical inactivity is a public health crisis which contributes to the development of many preventable diseases.

- Regular, planned exercise and other forms of physical activity are critical for overall health. Exercise improves health by reducing the risks for developing cardiovascular disease, type 2 diabetes mellitus, colon and breast cancer, obesity, depression and anxiety, and all-cause and premature mortality.

- Exercise is used as a treatment method for many diseases including cardiovascular, pulmonary, metabolic, and neurological diseases.

- Regular exercise can help college students achieve academic success and avoid contracting the common cold.

References

1. Boyle, J. P., Thompson, T. J., Gregg, E. W., Barker, L. E., & Williamson, D. F. (2010). Projection of the year 2050 burden of diabetes in the US adult population: Dynamic modeling of incidence, mortality, and prediabetes prevalence. *Popular Health Metrics, 8*(29), 1–12.

2. Center for Disease Control and Prevention. (2017, April 10). National Center for Chronic Disease Prevention and Health Promotion, Division of Nutrition, Physical Activity and Obesity, Atlanta, GA. Retrieved from https://www.cdc.gov/nccdphp/dnpao/data-trends-maps/index.html (accessed May 11, 2017).

3. Garber, C. E., Blissmer, B., Deschenes, M. R., Franklin, B. A., Lamonte, M. J., Lee, I. M., Nieman, D. C., & Swain, D. P. (2011). American College of Sports Medicine position stand. Quantity and quality of exercise for developing and maintaining cardiorespiratory, musculoskeletal, and neuromotor fitness in apparently healthy adults: Guidance for prescribing exercise. *Medicine and Science in Sports and Exercise, 43*(7), 1334–1359.

4. Hallal, P. C., Andersen, L. B., Bull, F. C., Guthold, R., Haskell, W., Ekelund, U., & Lancet Physical Activity Series Working Group. (2012). Global physical activity levels: Surveillance progress, pitfalls, and prospects. *Lancet, 380*(9838), 247–257.

5. Selvin, E., Parrinello, C. M., Sacks, D. B., & Coresh, J. (2014). Trends in prevalence and control of diabetes in the United States, 1988–1994 and 1999–2010. *Annals of Internal Medicine, 160*(8), 517–525.

6. Warburton, D. E., Katzmarzyk, P. T., Rhodes, R. E., & Shephard, R. J. (2007). Evidence-informed physical activity guidelines for Canadian adults. *Applied Physiology, Nutrition, and Metabolism, 32*(S2E), S16–S68.

Image Credits

- 1.1: Copyright © Depositphotos/leetorens.

- 1.2: Copyright © Depositphotos/ArturVerkhovetskiy.

- 1.3: Copyright © Depositphotos/Wavebreakmedia.

- 1.4: Copyright © Depositphotos/cupertino.

- 1.5: Kole E. Carpenter, "USS Nimitz Holds a Weightlifting Competition," https://commons.wikimedia.org/wiki/File:USS_ Nimitz_holds_a_weightlifting_competition._(10350108455).jpg. Copyright in the Public Domain.

- 1.6: Copyright © Depositphotos/SimpleFoto.

- 1.7: Rhoda Baer, "Senior Man in Gym," https://commons.wikimedia. org/wiki/File:Nurse_poses_with_cancer_patient.jpg. Copyright in the Public Domain.

- 1.8: Copyright © Ranveig (CC by 2.0) at https://commons.wikime-dia.org/wiki/File:Man_Flu.jpg.

- 1.9: Copyright © Depositphotos/Pixelchaos.

- 1.10: Copyright © Depositphotos/pressmaster.

- 1.11: Copyright © Depositphotos/photographee.eu.

HEALTH-RELATED COMPONENTS OF PHYSICAL FITNESS

I lift weights four times per week so I will be healthy.

Why should it matter what type of exercise I do?

As previously discussed, there is a distinct difference between physical activity and exercise. Physical activity is broadly defined as any bodily movements resulting in a notable increase in the calories being burned to fuel the activity. Playing a pickup game of basketball, taking in a round of golf, going on a leisurely stroll through a local metro park, and performing a strenuous job task such as mowing the lawn are all examples of physical activity. Health professionals harp on the value of getting more physical activity as doing so helps ward off many chronic and preventable diseases.

While physical activity is highly beneficial for improving health, physical activity in and of itself is not exercise. Exercise provides the biggest "bang for our buck" in terms of improving health. Exercise differs from physical activity based on a person's intent. That is, in order to exercise, a conscious effort needs to take place in a planned and orchestrated manner with the goal of improving physical fitness. It is through improvements in physical fitness that health benefits are best achieved!

Physical fitness is one of the most powerful predictors of health, disease risk, and premature mortality. Given the criticality of physical fitness on health, this chapter hones in on the topic of physical fitness. Specifically, this chapter focuses on the health-related components of physical fitness, how regular exercise influences these components, and how the components of health-related fitness play a role in overall health and disease risk.

2.1: What Is Fitness? Health-Related and Skill-Related Fitness

Fitness refers to a state of being in good overall health as a result of regular exercise. Within the discussion of fitness are the terms physical fitness, health-related fitness, and skill-related fitness. Physical fitness can be defined as a set of characteristics people have or can achieve to enhance their ability to perform physical activity or exercise. These characteristics can be split into health and skill-related components. The skill-related components of physical fitness consist of agility, coordination, power, balance, reaction time, and speed (Table 2.1). Improvements in these components are necessary if the goal of an exercise program is to increase sport-specific performance. Additionally, improvements of these components can carry over to overall health by reducing the risk of falling or injury. For instance, people who have good balance and coordination may not fall, twist an ankle, or pull a muscle when unsuspectingly stepping into a pot hole. However, an in-depth discussion concerning the skill-related components of physical fitness is beyond the scope of this book. For more information on how to improve the skill-related components of physical fitness consider reviewing materials from the National Strength and Conditioning Association or the National Academy of Sports Medicine.

Table 2.1 Skill-Related Components of Fitness	
Agility	The ability to change direction quickly while the body is in motion. An example of agility is when a running back in football moves to evade a tackler.
Coordination	The ability to use the body's senses together with the body's limbs in order to perform movement tasks smoothly. An example of coordination is how a basketball player can dribble a basketball while running without looking down.
Power	The ability to exert a maximal force in the shortest amount of time as possible. An example of power is swinging a baseball bat in an attempt to hit a ball as far as possible.
Balance	The ability to maintain proper posture or equilibrium while the body is in motion or stationary. An example of balance is riding on a skateboard and not falling over.
Reaction Time	Refers to the time between initial stimulus to move and the actual movement. An example of reaction time is the time between the sound of the gun and a sprinter moving out of the starting blocks.
Speed	The ability to perform a task within a short amount of time. An example of speed is an athlete performing a 40-yard sprint.

Table 2.2 Health-Related Components of Fitness	
Cardiorespiratory Endurance	The ability of the cardiovascular and respiratory systems to supply oxygen-rich blood to working muscles during exercise. An example of cardiorespiratory endurance is a marathoner being able to continuously run throughout a race.
Muscular Strength	The ability of skeletal muscle to exert a maximal force. An example of muscular strength is a weight lifter being able to complete a record-setting bench press.
Muscular Endurance	The ability of skeletal muscle to continuously exert a force without fatigue. An example of muscular endurance is a wrestler warding off being pinned by elevating the shoulders off the mat.
Body Composition	Refers to the relative amounts of muscle, body fat, and bone. An example of body composition is maintaining 12% body fat.
Flexibility	The ability to move a joint throughout its full range of motion. An example of flexibility is a person being able to bend at the waist and touch the toes.

More important to overall health are the health-related components of physical fitness. For most people, the goal of an exercise program should be to improve one or more of these components. Doing so will have a measurable impact on health and the reduction of disease risk. These health-related components of physical fitness are cardiorespiratory endurance, muscular strength, muscular endurance, body composition, and flexibility (Table 2.2). The remaining focus of this chapter will be on the importance of the health-related components of physical fitness for maintaining good health, preventing disease, and how exercise plays a role in improving these components.

Cardiorespiratory Endurance

One of the most widely studied components of health-related physical fitness is cardiorespiratory endurance. In fact, research has identified a person's cardiorespiratory endurance to be one of the most powerful predictors for developing preventable diseases and dying prematurely! Cardiorespiratory endurance is defined as the maximal capacity of the cardiovascular and respiratory systems to supply oxygen-rich blood to working muscles coupled with the muscles' ability to extract and utilize oxygen from the blood during sustained physical activity. In human physiology (the study of human bodily functions), the process by which the heart, lungs, blood vessels, and muscles work in unison to transport oxygen from the outside air to muscles or other cells is called the oxygen transport system. Once

Jogging for Cardiorespiratry Endurance

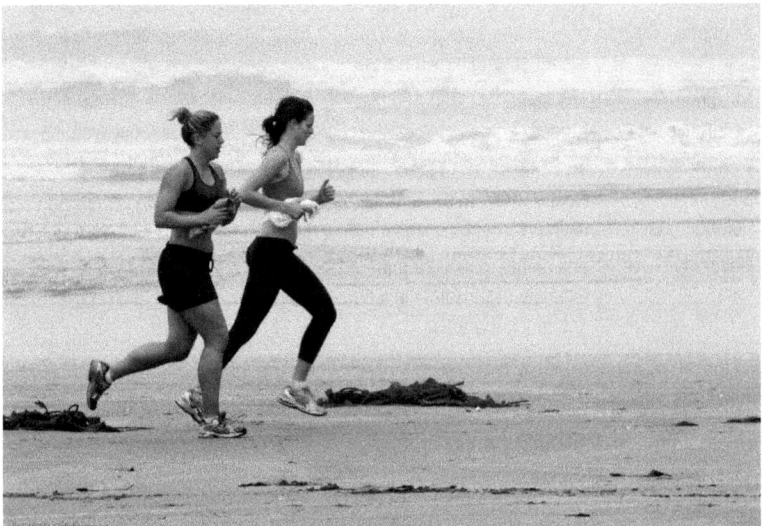

oxygen reaches the muscles or other cells, that oxygen is then used to build molecules needed to fuel muscular contractions or other cellular functions. Without adequate amounts of oxygen reaching the body's cells, with the exception of red blood cells, the cells will either lose proper function or die. Therefore, oxygen is essential to human survival and thus improvements in the capacity of the oxygen transport system are paramount in health and preventing disease.

The maximal capacity of the oxygen transport system (cardiorespiratory endurance) is measured by assessing VO_2max. VO_2max refers to the volume of oxygen that the body, especially the muscles, consume during exercise. The goal of any cardiorespiratory endurance exercise program should be, at a minimum, to improve VO_2max. Improving VO_2max is beneficial for many areas of health including improving heart and lung function, maintaining or losing body fat, preventing atherosclerotic plaque buildup in the arteries, maintaining healthy levels of blood glucose and cholesterol, and even warding off cancer. Additionally, improving VO_2max results in an increased ability to exercise harder and therefore make better gains toward accomplishing long-term exercise goals (e.g., weight loss or running a marathon). Exercises that improve VO_2max and cardiorespiratory endurance are called aerobic exercises. The word aerobic means with oxygen. Since the cardiovascular and respiratory systems are at the center of the oxygen transport system, any exercise that is continuous, rhythmic in movement, and elevates heart rate and respiration over a prolonged period of time is considered aerobic exercise. Examples of aerobic exercises are walking, jogging, swimming, and cycling.

YOUR TURN 2.1

Improving Cardiorespiratory Endurance

Directions: Now that you know that any exercise which is continuous, contains rhythmic and repeated movements, and elevates heart rate and breathing over a prolonged period of time is considered aerobic exercise, list five aerobic exercises that you could do to improve cardiorespiratory endurance. Please do not include walking, jogging, swimming, or cycling as these were mentioned in the text. Feel free to be creative! Not all aerobic exercises have to take place in a gym or on a piece of exercise equipment! Then briefly explain why each exercise would be considered an aerobic exercise. Lastly, explain how improving your cardiorespiratory endurance could be beneficial to YOUR health (e.g., do you have a family history of heart disease and want to improve your cardiorespiratory endurance to reduce your personal risk?).

Aerobic Exercise	Why are these exercises considered aerobic?
How could improving cardiorespiratory fitness improve YOUR health?	

The Fick Equation describes how VO_2max is calculated. The Fick Equation explains that VO_2max is equal to maximal cardiac output x maximal a-vO_2 difference. Cardiac output refers to the amount of blood that is pumped out of the heart per minute. As oxygen-rich blood leaves the heart it travels throughout the body in blood vessels called arteries to working muscles and other cells. After the muscles and cells extract oxygen from the blood, the blood is then returned to the heart in blood vessels called veins. Since muscles and other cells extract oxygen from the blood, there is more oxygen in the blood in arteries as opposed to veins. This difference between the amount of oxygen in the arteries and in the veins is called the a-vO_2 difference. During exercise the heart beats more frequently and the muscles extract more oxygen to fuel the exercise, therefore both cardiac output and a-vO$_2$ difference increase during exercise.

With knowledge of the Fick Equation it can be understood how exercise improves VO$_2$max in one of two ways. One is by increasing the amount of oxygen that muscles extract from the blood during exercise which increases the a-vO$_2$ difference. However, for most people, the muscles do a very good job of extracting oxygen from arterial blood and, without blood doping (infusion of more red blood cells), there is generally an upper limit to the maximal a-vO$_2$ difference. The difference between the oxygen in the arteries and the veins usually maxes out at around 20 percent. Therefore, in young healthy people, VO$_2$max is most influenced by cardiac output.

Cardiac output is equal to heart rate x stroke volume. Stroke volume is defined as the amount of blood pumped from the heart each beat. During exercise, both heart rate and stroke volume increase. What is more, both heart rate and stroke volume increase with every increase in exercise intensity. This means the harder the exercise, the higher the heart rate and stroke volume will be. However, heart rate has a physiological maximum which is largely dependent on age (i.e., 220 − age = max heart rate). Therefore, it is the maximal stroke volume that ultimately determines when young healthy people reach their VO$_2$max.

When examining the stroke volume response to aerobic exercise one finds that the stroke volume increases with each additional increase in exercise intensity. Unfortunately, for non-elite aerobic conditioned athletes, stroke volume maxes out at around 60 percent of a person's VO$_2$max. This means in order to significantly improve VO$_2$max, stroke volume must be higher at the point it maxes out. For most people, stroke volume maxes out at around 130 milliliters per heartbeat. With regular aerobic exercise maximal stroke volume can be significantly improved beyond 130 milliliters per beat and therefore increase VO$_2$max.

Improvement of VO$_2$max is paramount in achieving heart health. Not only does regular exercise improve maximal a-vO$_2$ difference and stroke volume, it also improves the a-vO$_2$ difference and stroke volume at rest. Such improvements lead to lower resting heart rates; less strain on the heart; lower blood pressure; optimal levels of glucose, fat, and cholesterol in the blood; and ultimately less atherosclerotic plaque buildup in the arteries. These improvements go a long way in increasing overall health and in preventing many chronic diseases. Consider "VO$_2$max and Your Health" to gain a better understanding of how increasing cardiorespiratory endurance improves health and wards off disease.

SUPPLEMENT YOUR LEARNING 2.1

VO_2max and Your Health

Improvement of VO_2max is indicative of an increased capacity and efficiency of the oxygen transport system. The oxygen transport system consists of the lungs, heart, blood vessels, and skeletal muscles and other cells, all of which work together to get oxygen from the air we breathe to the site of working muscles and cells. In the muscles and other cells, oxygen acts as a final receptor for electrons at the end of a series of many complex chemical reactions. This series of reactions, consisting of the breakdown of the foods we eat, leads to the construction of small molecules. It is these small molecules that are used to sustain the life and function of cells and to permit continued muscular contractions during exercise. Enhancements in the capacity and efficiency of the oxygen transport system result in numerous health benefits.

Coronary Artery Disease

Coronary artery disease is the most common cardiovascular disease and is responsible for the most deaths resulting from cardiovascular disease. Coronary artery disease results from the buildup of atherosclerotic plaque in the coronary arteries. Atherosclerotic plaque consists of fatty materials and LDL cholesterol in the blood which hardens and blocks the flow of blood through blood vessels. At rest and during exercise the muscles and cells need energy from the food we eat (fats, carbohydrates, and proteins). An improvement in the capacity and efficiency of the oxygen transport system permits the uptake of more fats and LDL cholesterol from the blood to be used for energy in the muscles and cells. Therefore, there is a decrease in the available fats and LDL cholesterol in the blood that can build up in the arteries of the heart.

Obesity

Obesity is marked by an abnormally high level of fat mass. As a result of regular aerobic exercise, the skeletal muscles adapt by increasing the amount oxygen they consume (increased a-vO$_2$ difference) and thereby increasing the amount of fat they can use for energy. By improving the oxygen transport system, muscles will use more fat for energy which helps in the reduction of body fat.

Type 2 Diabetes

Type 2 diabetes results from the inability of the skeletal muscles to react to insulin and pull in glucose from the blood. One way in which type 2 diabetes can occur is due to an accumulation of fats within skeletal muscle. This fat, called intramuscular triglycerides, interferes with the process of glucose uptake. As discussed above, improvements in the oxygen transport system result in an increase in fat use in skeletal muscle. Therefore, improving VO$_2$max helps reduce the amount of fat deposits in skeletal muscle and thereby prevent the interference of fat deposits on glucose uptake from the blood.

Cancer

Cancer is a highly complex set of diseases. The prevailing theory of cancer development suggests that cancer is caused by damage to DNA within the cells. As a result of damaged DNA the code for the reproduction of cells is compromised leading to the uncontrolled division of abnormal cells. Free radicals (electrons) can damage DNA. As previously mentioned, oxygen acts as a final receptor for electrons in the oxygen transport system to construct the small molecules needed to sustain the life and function of cells. By improving the efficiency of the oxygen transport system, there are more electrons binding to oxygen. This means that there will be less free radicals available to damage DNA. Therefore, improving VO$_2$max can help decrease the likelihood of developing cancer.

Since VO$_2$max is a major factor in health, it is important that cardiorespiratory endurance (aerobic) exercise be included in all exercise programs. Simply lifting weights a few times per week will not provide all of the health benefits needed. Designing a good exercise program for health will be covered in Chapter 4.

Muscular Strength

Muscular strength is defined as the ability of skeletal muscle to exert force and overcome an outside resistance. Consider the bench press. As people push on the barbell they exert a force and overcome the resistance of the weight loaded on the barbell. Improving or maintaining optimal muscular strength is very important for overall health. Long-term research suggests an inverse relationship between muscular strength and all-cause mortality. This means that as muscular strength decreases there is an increase in the risk for all-cause mortality. Alternatively, an increase in muscular strength reduces the risk of all-cause mortality. Muscular strength is associated with lower risks for developing cardiovascular diseases and many other chronic diseases. Additionally, muscular strength is associated with preserving muscle function and independence with age. Exercise aimed at increasing muscular strength can also reduce the risk for injury by subsequently increasing the strength of tendons and ligaments.

Aside from people who are deconditioned or suffering from various ailments, the only way to increase muscular strength is by performing resistance training. Resistance training involves performing a series of exercises in which the muscles contract against an external force or resistance. Examples of resistance training exercises include the bench press, squat, push press, and even planks.

There are four types of muscle contractions that can occur with resistance training. Most people are likely familiar with dynamic muscle contraction. A dynamic muscle contraction is an action that leads to movement of a given joint. The bench press, squat, and push press are examples of exercises that involve dynamic muscle contractions. Within dynamic muscle contractions there are two other subsets of contractions. The first of these contractions is called concentric muscle contraction. Concentric muscle contraction occurs when muscles shorten and cause the movement of a joint. Using the example of a biceps curl, the biceps shorten and pull the radius and ulna (lower arm bones) closer to the humerus (upper arm). The second contraction within dynamic muscle contractions is called eccentric muscle contraction. Eccentric muscle contraction occurs when muscles lengthen throughout a given movement and often occur when muscles have to slow down momentum. Using the example of a bench press, during the "down phase" the pectoral muscles lengthen and act to slow the weight from crashing down on the lifter's chest. Also, eccentric muscle contractions occur during downhill walking in order to slow down momentum. Lastly, there are isometric muscle contractions. Isometric muscle contractions occur when the muscle exerts a force but with no movement of a joint. An example of an isometric contraction is the action of the abdominal muscles during a plank. Here, the abdominal muscles contract in order to hold the abdomen off the ground, however there is no movement of a joint. Another example of an isometric contraction is when a person pushes hard against an immovable force such as a concrete wall. A resistance exercise program that incorporates all of these muscular actions has the capacity to increase muscular strength through several different mechanisms.

YOUR TURN 2.2

Improving Muscular Strength

Directions: Now that you know muscular strength can be increased by designing a resistance training program which incorporates the four types of muscle contractions, please list two resistance exercises for each type of muscle contraction. Then briefly explain why each of these exercises would lead to that type of contraction. Lastly, explain how improving muscular strength could be beneficial to YOUR health (e.g., do you have a history of certain injuries and want to reduce your future risk of more injuries?).

Resistance Exercise	Why does this exercise cause this type of contraction?
Dynamic Muscle Contraction:	
1.	
2.	
Concentric Muscle Contraction:	
1.	
2.	

Resistance Exercise	Why does this exercise cause this type of contraction?
Eccentric Muscle Contraction:	
1.	
2.	
Isometric Muscle Contraction:	
1.	
2.	
How could improving muscular strength improve YOUR health?	

The greatest factor for improving muscular strength is muscular hypertrophy. Muscular hypertrophy occurs when skeletal muscle adds more proteins and gets larger. Resistance exercise training is a powerful stimulus for muscular hypertrophy. In order for muscular hypertrophy to take place intramuscular proteins (proteins in the muscle cells) need to be continuously broken down and built back up. Resistance exercises act to break down intramuscular proteins. So when people perform a bench press they are breaking down proteins in the pectoral muscles. However, the muscles need time to recover and build up the proteins that are broken down during exercise. This is why it is never recommended to resistance train the same muscle group two days in a row. Of the different muscle contractions, all types can lead to muscular hypertrophy, but it is eccentric muscular contractions that cause the most damage to intramuscular proteins. So it can be said that exercises which emphasize eccentric contractions lead to more muscular hypertrophy. Not to be overlooked, however, is the impact of the nervous system on increases in muscular strength. Rather than being attributable to muscular hypertrophy, initial increases in muscular strength are mainly due to adaptations

Muscular Strength Training for Hypertrophy

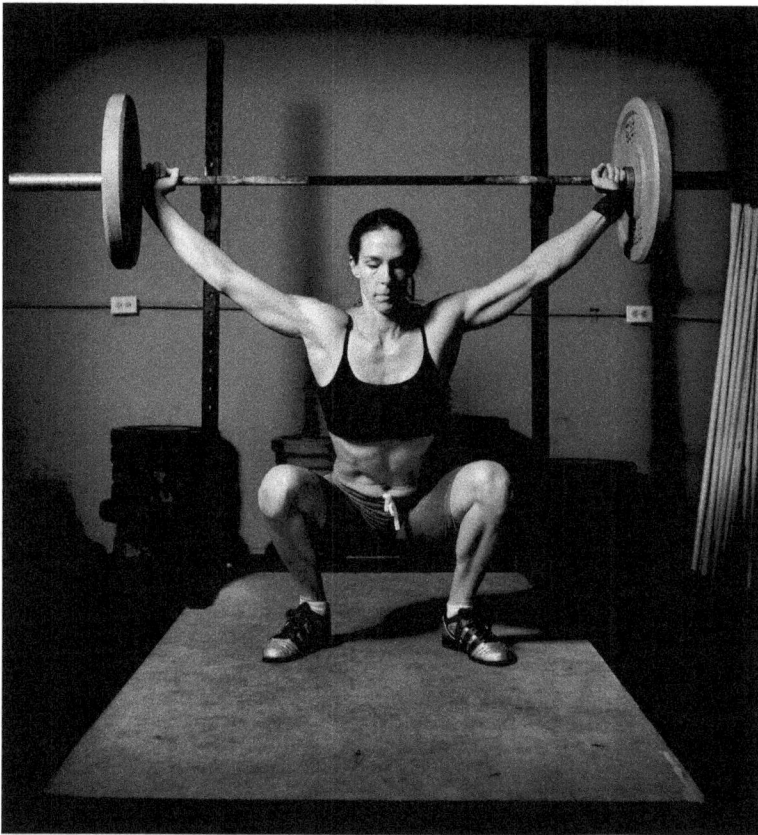

of the nervous system where more muscle fibers within the muscle are stimulated.

Stronger muscles are beneficial for overall health and the ability to do day-to-day activities. While resistance training alone is not sufficient for overall health, it is an important component and should be included in the exercise program design.

Muscular Endurance

Muscular endurance is often an overlooked component of health-related physical fitness. This view can be seen as problematic, especially since the benefits of having optimal muscular endurance encompass many aspects of overall health. These benefits include weight loss, maintaining a healthy body weight, more calories being burned at rest, lower blood pressure and blood lipids, enhanced glucose uptake, and a reduced risk of injury. Furthermore, completing an exercise program aimed at improving muscular endurance can lead to muscular hypertrophy, especially in people who are sedentary. Unlike muscular strength which is the ability of skeletal muscle to exert force, muscular endurance is defined as the ability of skeletal muscle to exert force over a period of time without fatigue. For instance, being able to do 100 push-ups in a row demonstrates good muscular endurance.

Similar to muscular strength, the best way to improve muscular endurance is by resistance training. The difference between resistance training for improving muscular endurance as opposed to muscular strength is the repetition scheme. In order to improve muscular strength, resistance exercises are performed with relatively more weight or resistance and lower repetitions. Muscular endurance, on the other hand, is improved when resistance exercises are performed with relatively less weight or resistance and more repetitions or time. Taking this into account, if people are trying to increase the muscular endurance of their pectoral muscles they may perform the bench press with a high number of repetitions or do many push-ups. Additionally, muscular endurance resistance training exercises can use body weight as the resistance. Examples of such exercises include push-ups, body squats, and crunches.

YOUR TURN 2.3

Improving Muscular Endurance

Directions: Now that you know muscular endurance, like muscular strength, is increased by doing resistance exercises and that the difference between the two is weight and repetition schemes, please list five resistance exercises aimed at increasing muscular endurance. Then briefly explain how the weight and repetitions are different for each exercise if you want to increase muscular strength. Lastly, explain how improving muscular endurance could be beneficial to YOUR health (e.g., do you want to lose weight?).

Resistance Exercise	How would the weight and repetition scheme change for increasing muscular strength?
1.	
2.	
3.	
4.	
5.	
How could improving muscular endurance improve YOUR health?	

People often train to improve their muscular endurance as a way to meet weight loss or aesthetic goals (e.g., trying to get a "six pack"). As for weight loss, repeatedly activating skeletal muscle through resistance exercise training increases the metabolic needs of skeletal muscle at rest. This means that skeletal muscles will burn more fats for fuel and ultimately more calories when a person is not exercising. In turn, this helps to reduce

Muscular Endurance Training Aids Weight Loss

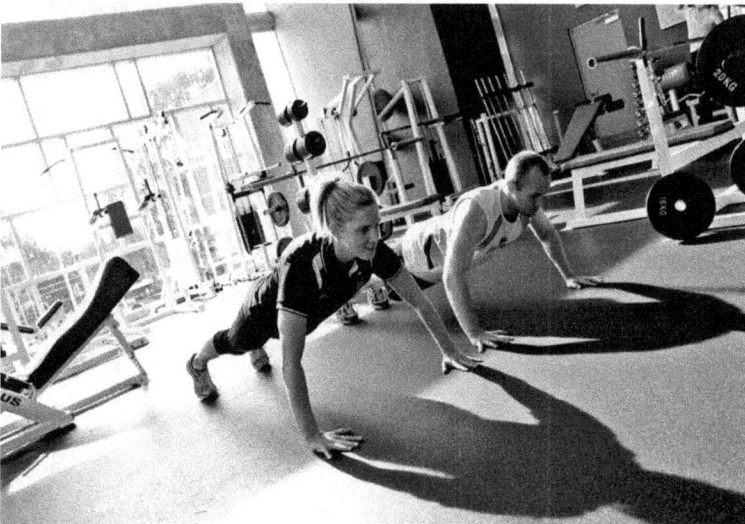

body weight and fat. Furthermore, the repeated muscular contractions that occur during resistance training induce the muscles to pull in more glucose from the blood during exercise and at rest. This acts to help people control their blood sugar which aids in the management and prevention of type 2 diabetes. Lastly, a common goal of many exercisers is to improve muscular tone. What this really means is people want to accentuate the appearance of their muscles. Training to improve muscular endurance helps accomplish this in two ways. The first is by eliciting weight loss and the second is through minor muscular hypertrophy.

The good news about improving muscular endurance is its relationship to muscular strength. Both are improved by resistance training exercises. However, the design of the program will determine how much strength versus endurance is improved. Generally a series of about 10 exercises that include 7 to 8 repetitions with curl-ups, planks, and push-ups or pull-ups provides good, balanced results. The specific design will be discussed in Chapter 4.

Monitoring Body Weight

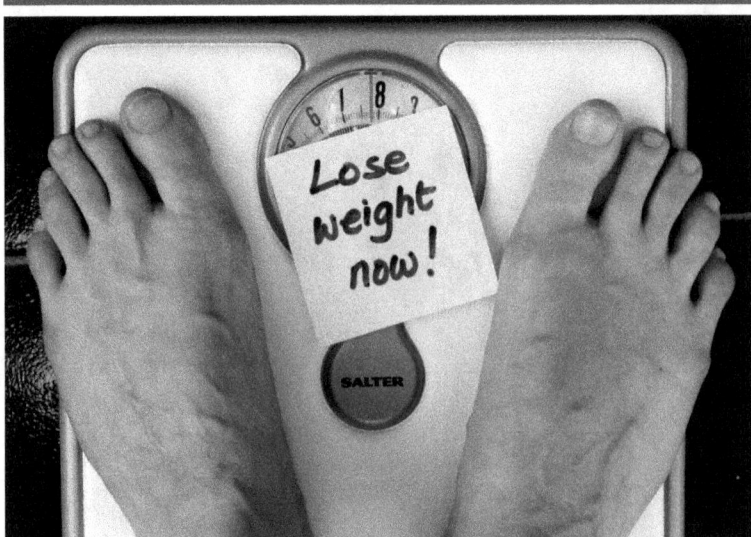

Body Composition

Body composition is a term that refers to the relative amounts of muscle, body fat, and bone in the human body. Most commonly, body fat is a highly stressed facet of body composition. However, not having enough muscle mass or bone density can lead to a plethora of negative health consequences. For instance, a loss of muscle mass leads to a loss of muscular strength which contributes to the majority of admissions into assisted living facilities. Also, a loss of bone density leads to osteoporosis and an increased risk for serious bone fractures. Beyond the physical consequences of living with poor body composition, there are mental and emotional consequences as well. Poor body composition is associated with depression, anxiety, and low self-esteem.

In the United States, poor body composition is a major public health concern, particularly when it comes to body weight and fat. Nearly two-thirds of adults in the United States are classified as overweight or obese.[2] Additionally, nearly 35 percent of all college students are classified as overweight or obese,[1] indicating that body composition is not just an issue for aging adults. For these individuals, the health risks are far reaching as high body weight and fat are associated with elevated risks for developing cardiovascular diseases, type 2 diabetes mellitus, and certain cancers.

Diet Plus Exercise is Best for Weight Loss

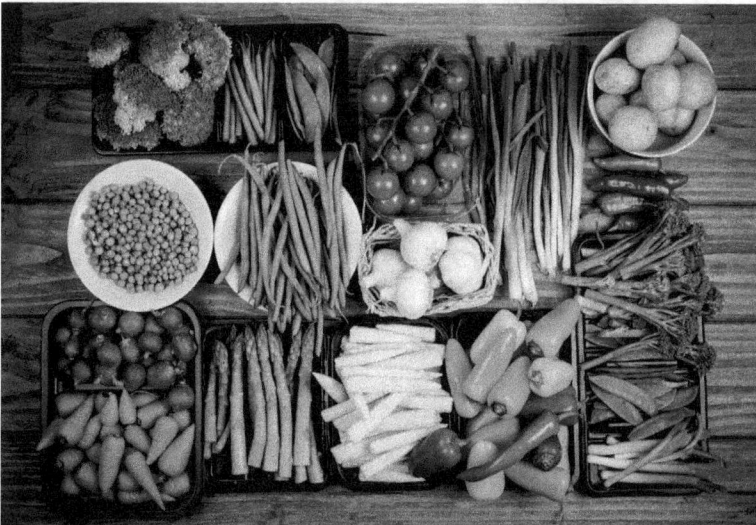

Having a proper diet is an excellent start for maintaining and achieving an appropriate body composition. For example, a well-rounded diet consisting of the proper calorie portions, macronutrients (carbohydrates, fats, and proteins), vitamins, and minerals will aid in maintaining or achieving a healthy weight and bone mineral content. However, proper diets work best when coupled with regular exercise. An example of this is the consumption of calcium-rich foods and bone mineral content. Simply eating calcium-rich foods does little in terms of improving bone mineral content. The bones must be stressed in order to uptake calcium. So without exercise, especially resistance exercises, calcium in calcium-rich foods will not be adequately absorbed by the bone. Diet and caloric restriction are paramount in losing weight; however, weight loss is best achieved and maintained when coupled with regular exercise.

Reductions in body weight and fat through regular exercise occur due to repeated elevations in resting metabolic rate. Resting metabolic rate represents the amount of calories burned when the body is at rest. Exercise influences resting metabolism through a variety of mechanisms. The main

High-Intensity Interval Training Can be Done on Machines

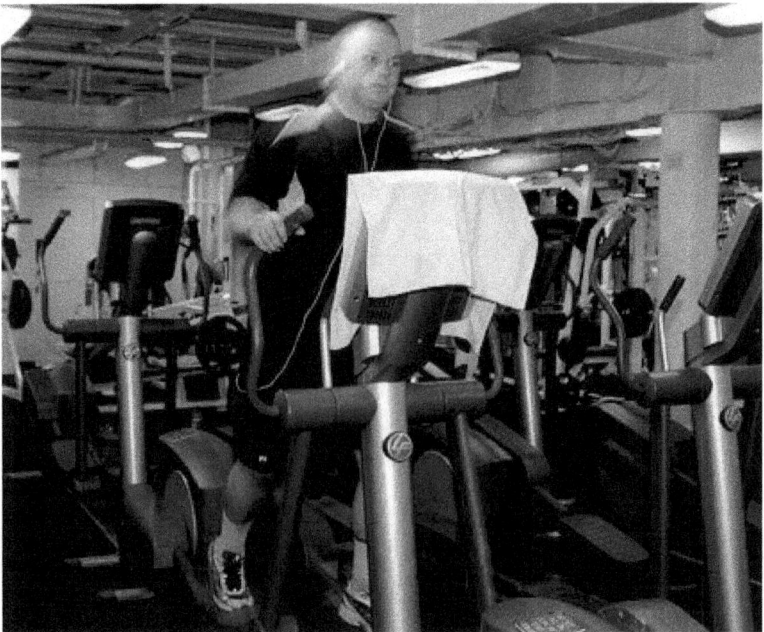

mechanism is the phenomenon known as excess post-exercise oxygen consumption. Excess post-exercise oxygen consumption represents the elevation of oxygen consumption up to 48 hours after exercise. This phenomenon results in more calories being burned at rest. Simply put, exercises that induce the greatest increase in excess post-exercise oxygen consumption will result in the most calories being burned at rest. Typically, these exercises are more challenging in nature such as high-intensity interval training.

Both aerobic and resistance exercise training can elicit positive changes in body composition. Overall, aerobic exercise is generally superior to resistance training for reducing body weight and fat. Resistance training, on the other hand, is generally better for increasing muscle mass and bone content. However, most researchers and health practitioners recommend an exercise program that contains both aerobic and resistance exercises to best improve or maintain an appropriate body composition.

Flexibility

The health-related benefits associated with improved flexibility have been the subject of much debate over the years. The term flexibility refers to a person's ability to move a given joint throughout its full range of motion. Some evidence suggests that regular flexibility exercise training can improve posture and balance. Other studies show that improvements in flexibility help reduce lower back and joint pain. However, as some studies that show

MYTH BOX: IDEAL BODY COMPOSITION ALWAYS EQUALS GOOD HEALTH AND HEALTHY OUTCOMES.

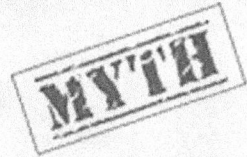

There is no question that maintaining a healthy body weight and body fat percentage is beneficial for overall health. A healthy weight and body fat percentage reduces the risks for developing cardiovascular diseases, type 2 diabetes, certain cancers, and dying at a premature age. As a result of this knowledge, coupled with the obesity epidemic, the diet industry has boomed. Expensive supplements, medications, surgeries, and nutrition plans are frequently used to help people reach an ideal body weight with less body fat. However, body weight and body fat in and of themselves are not the be-all and end-all for predicting healthy outcomes.

In fact, there have been several studies that evaluatated the likelihood of developing cardiovascular disease or dying prematurely in the presence of certain risk factors. These risk factors include obesity, high blood pressure, chronic illness, tobacco use, high cholesterol, and low cardiorespiratory fitness. Of these risk factors, low cardiorespiratory fitness (VO_2max) is the strongest predictor of cardiovascular disease and premature death! More importantly, people with high levels of cardiorespiratory fitness who smoke, have high blood pressure, have high cholesterol, and are obese have a lower risk for developing cardiovascular disease or dying prematurely than people who have none of these risk factors but have low levels of cardiorespiratory fitness. This means that having good cardiorespiratory fitness, even in the presence of other risk factors, is more predictive of good health outcomes than having no risk factors but having low cardiorespiratory fitness. Therefore, the take-away message is that even if regular exercise has little impact on your body weight, cholesterol, or blood pressure it still helps improve your cardiorespiratory fitness, which is the strongest predictor of healthy outcomes!

REFERENCES:

Barry, V. W., Baruth, M., Beets, M. W., Durstine, J. L., Liu, J., & Blair, S. N. (2014). Fitness vs. fatness on all-cause mortality: A meta-analysis. *Progress in Cardiovascular Diseases*, *56*(4), 382–390.

Blair, S. N., Kampert, J. B., Kohl, H. W., Barlow, C. E., Macera, C. A., Paffenbarger, R. S., & Gibbons, L. W. (1996) Influences of cardiorespiratory fitness and other precursors on cardiovascular disease and all-cause mortality in men and women. *JAMA, 276*(3), 205–210.

poor flexibility is associated with low back and joint pain others do not. What is clear is that improvements in flexibility are beneficial for sport-specific performance (e.g., being able to move the hip joint through a full range of motion when punting a football) and executing activities of daily living.

Flexibility varies from joint to joint and depends on a number of factors. Range of motion is limited by the configuration of bones, where bones fit together, and the properties of ligaments and muscles. For instance, the configuration of bones in the shoulder joints permit a wider range of motion compared to the configuration of bones in the knee joint. Muscles and ligaments can also limit range of motion. Muscles and ligaments can become tighter based on the stresses imposed on them. For example, sitting at a desk all day may result in the hip flexor muscles adapting to being a shorter length. They will therefore tighten, making it difficult to get into a proper upright position when standing. Additionally, exercise training can cause muscle adhesions and make movement a greater challenge. Flexibility exercise training improves range of motion by either passively or actively lengthening the muscles and ligaments.

Given that range of motion varies joint to joint, the focus of flexibility exercise training should be to improve the range of motion for each major muscle group. These groups consist of the hamstrings, quadriceps, glutes, calves, chest muscles, and back muscles. There are five main types of flexibility exercises: dynamic, static, ballistic, active, and passive exercises. Dynamic flexibility exercises involve the controlled movement of a joint through its full range of motion without holding the stretch in place (e.g., walking lunges). These flexibility exercises are best suited as a part of a warm-up for sporting events as they do not lead to reductions in sport performance. Static flexibility exercises consist of slowly stretching a muscle group and holding the stretch in place (e.g., sit-and-reach). These flexibility exercises are arguably the most commonly used exercises for increasing range of motion and work best following a light warm-up consisting of cardiorespiratory endurance exercises. Ballistic flexibility exercises use the body's momentum to increase the range of motion (e.g., bouncing up and down in attempt to reach the toes during a hamstring stretch). Ballistic stretching generally results in greater range of motion during a stretch than with dynamic or static flexibility exercises; however, ballistic stretches are generally not recommended as they have a tendency to lead to injury. Active stretching consists of holding a stretched muscle in place using the contraction of an opposite muscle group (e.g., contracting the hip flexors in order to hold a hamstrings stretch). Lastly, passive stretching takes place when a stretch is held in place by gravity, a device, or another person (e.g., partner stretching or stretching with bands).

The ability to move freely without pain is important for healthy living. All exercise programs should include a component of flexibility training. Choosing flexibility exercises is dependent upon a person's skill, fitness level, supervision, and available equipment. Generally, static stretching at the end of a regular workout a few times per week is recommended as a part of exercise programs aimed at improving health.

YOUR TURN 2.4

Improving Flexibility

Directions: Now that you know you should perform flexibility exercises for each of the major muscle groups in order to increase flexibility, list one flexibility exercise for each of these muscle groups. Then identify whether the flexibility exercise is a dynamic, ballistic, static, active, or passive. Lastly, explain how improving flexibility could be beneficial to YOUR health (e.g., do you have low back pain?).

Flexibility Exercise	Identify the type of flexibility exercise (dynamic, ballistic, static, active, or passive)
Hamstrings (back of upper leg):	
1.	
Quadriceps (front of upper leg):	
1.	
Glutes (buttocks):	
1.	
Calves (back of lower leg):	
1.	
Chest:	
1.	
Back:	
1.	
How could improving flexibility improve YOUR health?	

VOICES FROM CAMPUS 2.1

Christina

My mom and dad both have type 2 diabetes and are classified as obese. Just last week my dad had a terrible pain in his chest and we called the ambulance. Waiting in the emergency room for word on his condition was very stressful. Thoughts of the worst ran through my head. After a couple hours of waiting in agony, the doctor came out and said my dad had a heart attack and that they placed a stent in one of his coronary arteries. The doctor then said my dad needs to see his cardiologist in a week to check on his progress. My dad is only 45 years old.

In the cardiologist's office, the cardiologist emphasized that my dad needs to exercise regularly to avoid having another heart attack. The cardiologist then turned her attention to me. She told me that I need to start exercising because my mom and dad are obese, have type 2 diabetes and my dad just had a heart attack and those diseases run in the family. She then told me I need to start exercising now so that I don't become overweight, get type 2 diabetes, and have heart disease at a young age.

I took my dad's cardiologist's advice to heart, literally, and went to the gym the first thing the next day. This was the first time I had ever been in a gym and I was confused as to what I should be doing. So I talked to one of the gym's trainers and he got me started. He told me that I should emphasize aerobic exercise so I can increase my cardiorespiratory endurance as this would best reduce my risk for heart disease. He told me aerobic exercises are those where you continuously move and make your heart beat faster and make you breathe harder. He also told me I should do some resistance exercises to increase my muscular endurance because these exercises would help me burn more calories at rest which can keep me from gaining weight.

Now I exercise regularly and am doing great! I do aerobic exercises like the elliptical and stationary bicycle for 30 minutes per day, three days per week. I also do 50 push-ups, 100 body squats, 150 crunches, 25 walking lunges, 30 dumbbell push presses, and 30 supine pull-ups two days per week. In addition, I stretch after every workout to avoid getting tight muscles. I am now in the best shape of my life. The trainer at the gym tells me I now have an above average VO_2max for my age, that I have 18 percent body fat, and that if I keep it up I am far less likely to have heart disease or type 2 diabetes. My advice to any college student is to start moving more! You will feel great and you get healthier!

2.2: The Take Away

- Regular exercise is the best way to improve physical fitness and it is through improvements in physical fitness that health benefits are best achieved!

- Physical fitness is subdivided into health- and skill-related components. The health-related components of physical fitness are cardiorespiratory endurance, muscular strength, muscular endurance, body composition, and flexibility.

- An exercise program aimed at improving health should, at the very least, target improvements in one or more of the components of health-related physical fitness.

- Cardiorespiratory endurance level (VO_2max) is the strongest predictor for disease and premature death. Ideally, an exercise program aimed at improving health should incorporate some aerobic exercises to increase VO_2max.

- Exercising to improve any of the health-related components of physical fitness has a carryover effect on certain aspects of health. For instance, exercising to increase cardiorespiratory endurance can have a positive influence on body weight management and disease risk. Exercising to increase flexibility, on the other hand, has little impact on body weight management but can have a positive effect on pain.

- A person must identify specific goals for exercise and select aerobic, resistance, or flexibility exercises that can best accomplish those goals.

References

1. American College Health Association. (2013, spring). National college health assessment II: Undergraduate students: Reference group executive summary. Hanover, MD: American College Health Association.
2. Center for Disease Control and Prevention. (2017, April 10). National Center for Chronic Disease Prevention and Health Promotion, Division of Nutrition, Physical Activity and Obesity, Atlanta, GA. Retrieved from https://www.cdc.gov/nccdphp/dnpao/data-trends-maps/index.html (accessed May 11, 2017).

Image Credits

PRINCIPLES OF EXERCISE PROGRAM DESIGN

I go to the rec center to work out and just do what I feel like doing that day. Why does it matter what exercises I choose to do?

Thus far, several topics have been introduced. This book has discussed the difference between physical activity and exercise and how regular exercise can influence overall health. Additionally, it has been emphasized that through improvements in physical fitness, particularly the health-related components of physical fitness, better health outcomes are achieved. Also, aerobic, resistance, and flexibility exercise training have been discussed. Now the focus of this book will turn to the instruction of exercise program design.

Chapter 3 will build on the knowledge of the health-related components of physical fitness along with aerobic, resistance, and flexibility exercise training by introducing the basic principles of exercise program design. Here, individualization, SMART goals, and the principles of specificity, progressive overload, reversibility, and overtraining will be discussed. It is through an understanding and application of these concepts and principles that the health- and skill-related components of physical fitness can be improved. The road from the initiation of an exercise program to the realization of a healthier life begins with establishing baseline goals. To achieve these goals, an INDIVIDUALIZED exercise program must be implemented.

3.1: The Importance of Individualization

As previously discussed, exercise is the planned, structured, and repetitive application of physical activity (aerobic, resistance, or flexibility exercise training) with the goal of improving or maintaining one or more components of physical fitness. To improve any of the components of physical fitness, the body and its physiological systems must adapt to the exercise training. The principle of adaptation lies at the center of any exercise program. This principle states that if a specific physiological system is stressed on a consistent basis then that system will usually increase its capacity. For instance, if the cardiovascular system is regularly stressed by aerobic exercise training it will adapt by increasing the amount of blood pumped per beat at rest and during exercise.

Taking into account the principle of adaptation, it is imperative that an exercise program design be based on INDIVIDUAL health and fitness needs and goals. There is not a single exercise program that will benefit everyone in the same manner. Exercise programs should be different for different people. To put this into context, think of a visit to the doctor's office. Two people visit the doctor on the same day because they are both suffering from the signs and symptoms of an upper respiratory tract infection. However, the prescribing physician may prescribe an antibiotic for one patient but not the other. The reason is that while the signs and symptoms may be similar, one patient may have a bacterial infection while the other may have a viral infection. Giving these two patients the same medication may offer benefits to both patients; however, one would benefit markedly less. Carrying this example over to an exercise program design, two people may both be at an elevated risk for developing cardiovascular disease but one person may have dyslipidemia and the other may be obese. These two people would certainly benefit from the same exercise program design, but one person, perhaps the person who is obese, may not lose as much weight as needed.

Exercise programs are the most effective when they are individualized. First and foremost, exercise programs should be tailor made to suit a person's health and physical fitness goals. If a person's physical fitness goal is to lose weight, it makes little sense to design an exercise program consisting of solely resistance and flexibility training. Additionally, if a person's goal is to increase muscular strength, it makes little sense to design an exercise program that focuses mainly on aerobic exercise training. (See Voices From Campus 3.1 for an example of how to take into account individual health and fitness goals when designing an exercise program.)

Secondly, a person's health needs must be taken into account when designing an exercise program. While goals are extremely important when designing an exercise program, the program must address a person's health needs. Current diseases and risk factors for chronic disease development need to be taken into account because exercise impacts diseases and risk factors differently. To put this into context, consider two people: one person with type 2 diabetes and another who is obese and needs to lose weight. If a person has type 2 diabetes and is seeking to manage the disease through exercise, the exercise program needs to consist of exercise sessions separated by no more than two days of rest. The reason for this is that after an exercise session the skeletal muscles will increase glucose uptake from the blood for up to 48 hours post exercise. Therefore, to manage type 2 diabetes and keep blood glucose levels within an acceptable range there should not be more than a 48-hour period of physical inactivity. With the person who needs to lose weight there needs to be a constant caloric deficit. This means that over the course of a week a person needs to burn more calories than consumed. It is beneficial for people seeking to lose weight to exercise more frequently than if they are merely trying to control blood glucose levels. In this context, the point becomes clear that an exercise program must address a person's health needs.

Further, exercise programs must take into account a person's health and exercise history, age, likes and dislikes, physical limitations, past medical history, and current fitness level. Looking at exercise history is important when designing an exercise program—if a person has previously only exercised on the stationary bicycle and then suddenly starts exercising on the treadmill, the person will initially struggle and may not get the most out of the new exercise. This happens because the human body adapts based on the stresses imposed upon it. Therefore, someone who only cycles will not be as efficient on the treadmill. Additionally, physical limitations play a role in exercise selection. A person with chronic low back pain may not be able to do weight-bearing exercises to the same extent as someone without chronic back pain. Next, age comes into play when designing an exercise program. Exercise, particularly aerobic exercise, is prescribed based on age-predicted max heart rate (discussed in detail in Chapter 4). As people age maximal heart rate declines due to a loss of certain receptors in the heart. Therefore, a person who is 20 would have to exercise at higher heart rates to receive similar benefits as an older person. Next, current health status and past medical history must be considered. People respond differently to exercise when they have current or past ailments. Consider a person with chronic obstructive pulmonary disease. These people are limited in their exercise capacity due to a decreased ability to exhale air from the lungs. Therefore, exercise for people with chronic obstructive pulmonary disease needs to be less intense. After that, a person's current fitness level must be taken into account when designing an exercise program. The reason for this can be found in the law of initial value. Here, people with the lowest fitness levels will improve the most in comparison to those with higher initial fitness values. When designing an exercise program, the exercise intensity must be higher for those with higher fitness levels to improve; those with lower fitness levels can exercise at a lower intensity and they will still improve. Lastly, a person's likes and dislikes must be considered. The reason for this is fairly obvious, if a person does not like certain exercises he or she will not do them and may quit the exercise program. (See Voices From Campus 3.2 for an example of how to take into account a person's health and exercise history, current health status, age, likes and dislikes, physical limitations, past medical history, and current fitness level when designing an exercise program.)

VOICES FROM CAMPUS 3.1

Jameson

When I was 17 years old I tore the ACL in my right knee during my senior night high school football game. I was devastated as I was forced to miss the playoffs. In the midst of my injury, I was not able to do the exercises I once did and I was fairly depressed. So I stayed at home most nights, waited for my knee to heal, and ate a lot. As a result, I gained 35 pounds and became significantly overweight.

I am now a freshman in college and I realize I need to lose weight. However, I do not know what types of exercises would help me accomplish this goal. Additionally, my knee still hurts when I bear too much weight. In the past, my exercises were given to me by my football coach and I did them without question. I needed help, so I sought the advice of a fitness trainer at my college's recreation center.

The trainer told me that first I need to consider my individual goals. Given that my goal was to lose weight, the trainer said I should exercise most days of the week and do a combination of aerobic and resistance exercises. She explained that aerobic exercise burns the most calories during exercise and that resistance exercise helps me burn more calories at rest. To accommodate my knee pain, the trainer said I should do more non-load-bearing aerobic exercises like the stationary bike, rower, and swimming. For resistance exercises she suggested I do more machine-based exercises as they would allow me to control the weight more so than with free weights. After following her advice for two months my knee began to feel better and I lost eight pounds!

VOICES FROM CAMPUS 3.2

Wendy

I just started college this fall. I noticed that many of my classmates wear workout clothes to class and talk relentlessly about going to the gym. They take spinning, yoga, and Zumba classes at the recreation center. It appears they are in great shape and they have a lot of fun exercising. I have never really been physically active and am kind of a bookworm. I realize I need to be more physically active, after all I have read a lot about the freshman 15. I also think going to the gym regularly may help me make new friends.

The problem is I really don't like most exercises. I have tried cycling and aerobic classes back in high school and I absolutely hated them. I never felt so sore in my life. So I decided that before I hit the gym and give those spinning, yoga, and Zumba classes a go I needed to see a trainer.

The trainer told me my situation was more common than I thought. She began pressing me on physical activities that I enjoy. I stated that I really enjoyed playing squash in high school gym class. She informed me the rec center had squash courts and even had an open squash league three nights per week. She then said that I should take part in this open league as squash stresses the cardiorespiratory system and can help me avoid the freshman 15. She also said doing exercises and physical activities that I enjoy increases the likelihood I continue to exercise and that would even lead me to do even more exercise down the road. I took the trainer's advice and I now found out I really like the elliptical too. What's more is I even made new friends!

Goal Setting: SMART Goals

The first step in designing an effective exercise program is establishing baseline goals. If baseline goals are not established, designing an effective exercise program is extremely difficult. First off, baseline goals help determine the types of exercise training that should be done. For instance, if a person seeks to improve cardiorespiratory endurance, then that person would need to design an exercise program that consists of aerobic exercise training. Conversely, someone seeking to increase muscular strength would need to perform resistance exercise training.

Secondly, goals help people stay on track during their exercise training. Exercising aimlessly, while possibly beneficial, does little for pushing people toward optimal health. During the course of an exercise program people oftentimes plateau in their physical fitness. A lack of goals can result in the failure to overcome these plateaus. Thirdly, consider the principle of adaptation. Without establishing baseline goals it becomes incredibly difficult to properly stress the physiological systems needed to adequately improve overall health. The best strategy for establishing baseline goals for an exercise program is to set what are called SMART goals.

SMART is an acronym which contains the criteria for setting goals. The acronym stands for specific, measurable, achievable, relevant, and time-bound.

These criteria are used in many aspects of life. Business leaders, teachers, government officials, medical professionals, and everyday people use these criteria when setting goals. Setting SMART goals helps ensure short-term and long-term successes. In the area of exercise program design, the use of SMART goals is an excellent way to ensure that people get the absolute most out of exercise training. With that said SMART goals must be applied to exercise!

First the goal must be specific. Given this book is about exercising to improve health, the overreaching goal of improving health is far too vague. Improving health can be accomplished in many ways (e.g., improving one of the components of health-related physical fitness). Furthermore, it is extraordinarily challenging and likely impossible to design an exercise program which maximizes improvements to all components of health-related physical fitness. So it is important to pick a specific goal that will help improve health. For this an example would be weight loss. Here, the goal can be further specified to give a weight loss goal, like losing 20 pounds.

Secondly, goals must be measurable. If goals are not measurable, there is no quantifiable way to determine whether or not the exercise program is resulting in the physiological adaptations needed to meet a person's goals. Consider the vague goal of improving overall health. Aside from regular visits to the doctor's office, how would a person quantify improvements in health? This example drives home the point that goals must be quantifiable. With a goal like weight loss it is fairly easy to quantify and measure improvements. Here, tracking the loss of pounds would suffice nicely.

Thirdly, goals must be achievable. It is important to understand that for most people, becoming an elite marathoner, weight lifter, body builder, or even slimming down to 5 percent body fat are not achievable goals. All humans are limited by genetics. Some people have the genetics for achieving world class fitness status, but most people do not. This is not meant to be discouraging, it is simply being realistic. Goals like losing 20 pounds, completing a marathon, putting on muscle mass, and even getting a six pack are definitely achievable, but they require a significant effort and relentless discipline. While goals should be achievable, they should not be too easy to accomplish. Losing 5 pounds over a 20-week period may be far too easy since this goal may reasonably be achieved in 2 weeks. There needs to be some ambition driving the goals that are set.

Fourthly, goals need to be relevant to the person setting the goal. Meaning goals that are set by a third party may not necessarily be interpreted as relevant by the person receiving them. Consider a person who is obese. A third party may set this person a goal of running a 10K race. The person who is obese may not consider this goal all that important. After all, this person needs and likely wants to lose weight. While training to run a race like a 10K would likely result in weight loss, the person receiving the goal may not see this in the big picture and opt to quit an exercise program. Therefore, people should set goals that matter to them, leading to goals that are more likely to be achieved and more consistent adherence to an exercise program.

Lastly, goals need to be time-bound. This means that goals need to be made with specific end points in mind. An example of this would be losing 20 pounds in 20 weeks. Furthermore, long-term goals need to be broken into short-term goals. An example of this would be losing one pound per week over the course of an exercise program. Doing this helps keep people motivated and moving toward accomplishing their goals.

YOUR TURN 3.1

Setting SMART Goals

Directions: The SMART criteria for setting goals suggests that goals should be specific, measurable, achievable, relevant, and time-bound. Please list three SMART goals that you would have going into an exercise program. Then, for each goal briefly explain how the goal is specific, measurable, achievable, relevant to you, and time-bound.

Goal	How is the goal specific, measurable, achievable, relevant to you, and time-bound?
1.	S: M: A: R: T:

2.	S: M: A: R: T:
3.	S: M: A: R: T:

The Principle of Specificity

Now that goals have been established and things like a person's health needs, current health status, health and exercise history, physical limitations, age, likes and dislikes, and current fitness level have all been taken into account, it is time to start designing the actual exercise program. At this point, the objectives are to pick the type(s) of exercise training (aerobic, resistance, or flexibility training) and individual exercises to be completed in the exercise program. To meet these objectives, it is imperative to have an understanding of one of the most basic principles of exercise program design. This principle is called specificity.

The principle of specificity refers to exercise training that is carried out in a very specific manner intended to elicit a specific physiological adaptation. At the center of the principle of specificity is Wolff's Law. Wolff's Law suggests that the human body and its physiological systems will adapt to the stresses imposed. Extending Wolff's Law and specificity to exercise, the only way for a physiological system to adapt is by choosing exercises that stress that system.

To simplify this principle, consider the following three simple scenarios. If a person seeks to improve cardiorespiratory endurance, then aerobic exercises must be performed. If the goal is to increase muscular strength or endurance, then resistance exercises must be performed. If a person wants to improve flexibility, then flexibility exercises must be performed. Things do become a little bit more challenging when the goal of an exercise program is to improve a specific aspect of health. Here, it is important to consider the physiological systems that need to be stressed. For instance, for goals like the reduction of blood pressure, cholesterol, body weight, or blood sugar an exercise program that stresses both the cardiovascular and skeletal muscle systems work best. Please refer back to Chapters 1 and 2 to determine which physiological systems need to be stressed to achieve certain health goals.

YOUR TURN 3.2

Applying the Principle of Specificity

Directions: Now that you know that you need to select exercises that stress the specific physiological systems that align with your goals, please list five exercises for each goal you established in Your Turn 3.1. Then briefly explain how the exercises you chose stress the physiological system needed to accomplish your goals.

Goals	Exercises	How do these exercises stress the necessary physiological system?
1.	1.	
	2.	
	3.	
	4.	
	5.	

2.	1.	
	2.	
	3.	
	4.	
	5.	
3.	1.	
	2.	
	3.	
	4.	
	5.	

The Principle of Progressive Overload

At this point, goals have been established, needs and other factors have been considered, and the type(s) of exercise training and exercises required have been identified. Now it is necessary to discuss how an exercise program needs to change over time in order to elicit the physiological adaptations required to accomplish goals and meet needs. Throughout an exercise program the body gradually adapts in response to the exercise being performed. This means the body will become used to a given level of exercise and reach a physiological maximum for that amount of exercise. Things like cardiorespiratory fitness level, muscular strength, muscular endurance, flexibility, and muscle mass will eventually stall at a given level of exercise. The only way to adapt further and move closer toward accomplishing goals and health needs is to add to the existing level of exercise. This is the idea behind the principle of progressive overload. The principle of progressive overload suggests that in order for a physiological system to improve its capacity, it must be forced to adapt to an exercise stimulus that is above and beyond what it has previously experienced. To increase the exercise

MYTH BOX: BY EXERCISING A SPECIFIC MUSCLE GROUP YOU CAN REDUCE FAT IN THAT AREA.

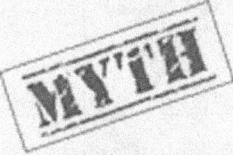

There is no doubt that exercising a specific muscle group can increase the size and efficiency of the muscles within that group. For instance, if people perform biceps curls three days per week, then they will see an increase in the size of the biceps. This is a great thing, after all who wouldn't want bigger biceps? However, problems may arise when people believe that exercising a specific muscle group will result in fat being burned from that area. A common perception many people have is that if they perform sit-ups all the time they will get a six pack. This is not the case! Doing sit-ups will definitely increase the size of the ab muscles, but fat will not be burned from that area.

When it comes to fat loss, the body does not liberate fat stores from the area of the body being trained. Consider a recent study[2] in which participants performed muscle endurance exercise using their non-dominant leg for 12 weeks. After that 12 weeks, the participants significantly reduced their total body fat mass.[2] However, the participants did not have a significant reduction in fat surrounding the exercised leg.[2] To put this into perspective, the fat surrounding muscle is not a property of that muscle.

stimulus imposed on a physiological system there are several changes that can be made to an exercise program. The first factor that is recommended is to increase the amount of time spent exercising. So if a person is exercising for 30 minutes per day, an increase to 35 minutes would add an additional exercise stimulus. The second method of progressive overload is by increasing the frequency of exercise. This is simply accomplished by exercising more days per week. Third, changes in the individual exercises can provide new and additional stimuli for continued improvement. The final method of progressive overload is to increase the exercise intensity. Increasing exercise intensity simply means to exercise harder. This can be accomplished by increasing the amount of weight being lifted or the speed and resistance of aerobic exercises. Usually increasing the exercise intensity should only be done once the time and frequency of exercise has been increased.

The Principle of Reversibility

While understanding the principles of specificity and progressive overload is critical in eliciting the physiological adaptations necessary for accomplishing goals and health needs, it is useful to understand what happens when an exercise program is stopped or delayed. A reduction in exercise training, whether by decreasing exercise frequency, time, or intensity, will result in the consequent loss of previously gained physiological adaptations. This process is known as detraining. Simply put, in order to keep exercise adaptations the level of exercise must remain at the same level as when the adaptations were gained. For instance, if a female student was running 30 minutes per day at a speed of 5 miles per hour, then she would need to continue this regimen to maintain her cardiorespiratory fitness level. Related to detraining is the principle of reversibility. The principle of reversibility suggests that the adaptations achieved through exercise are transient and can be lost once the stimulus of exercise is reduced or removed. This literally means "if you don't use it, you lose it!"

Improvements in muscle mass, strength and endurance, fat loss, flexibility, cardiorespiratory endurance, and other aspects of overall health are subject to being lost or reduced if an exercise program is delayed or terminated. The extent of these losses is largely dependent upon the length of time exercise has been reduced or ceased. Gains in muscular strength and muscle mass are lost fairly slowly after exercise has been stopped. Usually, noticeable reductions in muscular strength and muscle mass are seen after 12 weeks of inactivity. Improvements in cardiorespiratory endurance are lost more quickly than those of muscular strength and mass. Here noticeable declines in cardiorespiratory fitness level are seen after just two weeks of inactivity. The good news is that the physiological gains lost as a result of detraining can be re-gained more quickly than it originally took to achieve those gains in the first place. However, it is important to note that any delay or cessation of an exercise program will result in setbacks toward achieving goals and addressing health needs.

Therefore, contracting a certain muscle has no effect on the fat immediately outside the muscle.

During a bout of exercise, the fat from within a muscle is the first to be used for fuel.[1] As an exercise bout progresses, the body increases reliance on peripheral fat stores for fuel[1] (e.g., belly fat). Unfortunately, we have no control over where this peripheral fat comes from. This means that our body may break down peripheral fat stores from the legs, even though we may be doing sit-ups. In order to lose fat effectively, exercise durations should be increased and supplemented with days of resistance training. In short, losing weight and body fat is a slow process and requires dedication and attention to diet!

REFERENCES:

1. Horowitz, J. F., & Klein, S. (2000). Lipid metabolism during endurance exercise. *American Journal of Clinical Nutrition, 72*(2), 558s–563s.
2. Ramírez-Campillo, R., Andrade, D. C., Campos-Jara, C., Henríquez-Olguín, C., Alvarez-Lepín, C., & Izquierdo, M. (2013). Regional fat changes induced by localized muscle endurance resistance training. *Journal of Strength and Conditioning Research, 27*(8), 2219–2224.

Overtraining

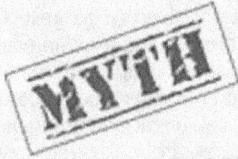

Exercise, in general, will improve something. Cardiorespiratory endurance, muscular strength, muscular endurance, body composition, and or flexibility will improve in response to any form of exercise or physical activity. However, meeting your goals or fitness and health needs requires a more detailed and scheduled approach to exercise training. Though any exercise is beneficial, simply doing the same exercises, at the same intensity, for the same amount of time will not help you meet goals. Consider Wolff's Law. Wolff's Law suggests that the body will adapt to the specific stresses imposed upon it. Thus, you will only improve to whatever level of exercise you do and little more! If you run 10 miles a day at 6mph, then you won't be able to run 10 miles at 7mph. If you want to lift 200 pounds but never lift more than 100 pounds, you will never meet your goal. You must implement overload into your exercise plan!

Successful exercise programs rely on the principle of progressive overload.[1] By gradually increasing exercise frequency, intensity, and time people move

Though it is necessary to implement the principle of progressive overload in an exercise program, it is important to not overdo it. A successful exercise program design involves the careful balancing act of progressive overload with adequate recovery time and rest. It is useful to understand that at the cellular level, exercise adaptations occur when proteins are broken down and built back up through protein synthesis. Exercise is the stimulus that causes the breakdown of proteins. During rest and recovery periods the proteins that were broken down during an exercise session are built back up. Repeating this process eventually leads to the physiological adaptations necessary for accomplishing goals and health needs. However, when overload becomes too excessive coupled with inadequate amounts of rest and recovery overtraining can occur.

Overtraining occurs when the amount of protein breakdown, as a result of exercise, exceeds the body's capacity to build those proteins back up. Overtraining leads to numerous negative consequences. The hallmark consequence of overtraining is a reduction in exercise capacity and performance. For instance, if someone was previously able to run for 45 consecutive minutes and all of a sudden has a hard time running just 20 consecutive minutes, that person may be overtraining. Other consequences of overtraining include the loss of physiological gains, chronic fatigue, increased perception of effort during light or moderate exercise, disturbed sleeping patterns, loss of appetite, and reoccurring illnesses such as the common cold. Once these symptoms occur it is critical that exercise be immediately reduced and rest days be increased so as to avoid further decrements in exercise capacity or physiological gains.

As a general rule, when applying the principle of progressive overload, exercise levels should not increase by more than 5 percent on a weekly basis. For instance, the exercise variables of frequency, intensity, and time should never be increased by more than 5 percent from one week to the other. Additionally, it is helpful to only increase one exercise variable at a time. Increasing all of the exercise variables at once is a recipe for overtraining, especially for new exercisers. For people just starting an exercise program, it is recommended that exercise time be increased first followed by frequency and then intensity.

steadily toward achieving their goals. It is recommended that either exercise frequency, intensity, or time be increased by approximately 5 percent from one week to the next. By doing this, the body is forced to adapt to greater stresses which leads to goal achievement. Furthermore, this modest increase in exercise stress permits the body ample time to adapt without overtraining. As a general rule of thumb, increase exercise frequency and time first before increasing exercise intensity.

REFERENCES:

1. Haff, G., & Triplett, N. T. (2015). *Essentials of strength training and conditioning* (4th ed.). Columbus, OH: Human Kinetics.

3.2: The Take Away

- Exercise provides stresses on the body that lead to physiological adaptations. The principle of adaptation explains that if a specific physiological system is stressed on a consistent basis, then that system will usually increase its capacity.

- The adaptations required to meet goals and health needs are most likely to occur if an exercise program is INDIVIDUALIZED.

- Exercise programs need to be individualized based on a person's goals, health needs, health and exercise history, age, likes and dislikes, physical limitations, past medical history, and current fitness level.

- Exercise program design begins with establishing goals. Goals should be specific, measurable, achievable, relevant, and time-bound (SMART).

- The principle of specificity suggests that the only way for a physiological system to adapt is by choosing exercises that stress that system.

- In order for a physiological system to continue to improve its capacity, exercise frequency, intensity, or time must be gradually increased. Exercise frequency, intensity, and time should be increased separately and should never be increased more than 5 percent from one week to the next.

- Any improvement achieved through exercise training can be lost once exercise is stopped or delayed. However, improvements can be re-gained more quickly after stopping an exercise program than at the onset of a new exercise program.

- Excessive overload can lead to overtraining. Overtraining can cause reductions in exercise capacity and performance.

- It is important to recognize the signs and symptoms of overtraining and immediately increase rest and recovery. Overtraining for prolonged periods results in significant delays in reaching goals.

DESIGNING AN EXERCISE PROGRAM

I want to stay healthy so I exercise. Why can't I just do what my friends do at the rec center?

A s previously discussed in Chapter 3, exercise goals must be established. This is best accomplished by using the SMART criteria: specific, measurable, achievable, relevant, and time-bound. This would include setting goals that are specific to the types of fitness improvements desired and measuring the changes in fitness over time.

In Chapter 4, SMART goals will be used to develop and monitor the progress of an exercise program. The first step is to assess the fitness level of the relevant components of health-related fitness and then develop a program to meet the intended goals. The "measurable" component of SMART goals is important to not only track the progress of the goals, but set initial exercise loads as well.

Purpose of Exercise Testing

In general, exercise testing serves two important functions in the design of an exercise program. First, it can help establish baseline information. In other words, exercise testing provides numerical scores for performance on fitness tests that can be used to determine the strengths and weaknesses of an individual's health and fitness. This information can then be used to design an effective exercise program to meet the individual's goals. Second, exercise testing is used to monitor progress toward achieving goals and how the exercise program may be changed over time in order to be more effective.

It is best to assess all of the components of fitness that are related to the individual's goals. The health-related components of fitness were described in Chapter 2 and should be considered when designing an exercise program for health. Some of the tests for cardiorespiratory fitness, muscular strength, muscular endurance, body composition, and flexibility will be discussed in this chapter.

Good fitness assessments must be done by a qualified fitness tester with appropriate fitness equipment. Many fitness centers, including those on college campuses, provide these assessments. There is generally a cost associated with this testing and it would be a good investment to get this information. However, the inability to get a formal fitness assessment should not stop someone from developing an exercise program. There are other ways to get started in exercise and track exercise progress. Most important is that the same testing procedures must be used each time the tests are repeated and compared!

4.1: Importance of Tracking Goals

Monitoring the progress of an exercise program is important in order to determine whether the program is working. One way to accomplish this is to periodically, every six months for example, complete an exercise assessment with a qualified tester, or at a minimum do a self-assessment as discussed in this chapter. The results of the tests over time will clearly show where improvements are being made and where more improvements are needed for each of the components of fitness tested. This information can

Figure 4.1 Sample Exercise Log

Date: _____Weight before exercise _____ lbs. Weight after exercise _____ lbs.

Exercises	Resistance				Cardio				
	Wt	Sets	Reps		Time	Dist	HR		

be used to modify the exercise program appropriately. Additionally, seeing the improvements made over time can be a powerful motivator to continue exercising for life!

While a good fitness assessment is ideal, goals can still be evaluated even if proper testing is not possible or costs too much for the budget. An option is to keep a detailed log of workouts. The distances covered on cardio machines and the amounts of weight lifted can show whether improvements are being made over time. It is also important to monitor body weight. Not only does it indicate whether weight is being gained or lost over the long term, it can help people determine how much water the body loses in the short term. (See Supplement Your Learning 4.1 Monitoring Hydration.). Specific examples for each component of health-related fitness will be provided later in the chapter. See Figure 4.1 for an example of an exercise log.

SUPPLEMENT YOUR LEARNING 4.1

Monitoring Hydration

Most people know about monitoring their body weight. They weigh themselves periodically to see if they lost or gained weight. This works well when performed over multiple days. However, the body weight fluctuates several pounds over the course of one day. These daily fluctuations are caused for the most part by body water changes. Since one pound of fat contains about 3500 calories, it is impossible to lose several pounds of fat in one day!

Water is the most important nutrient humans consume. It makes up over half of the body weight. Therefore, it is important to keep the body well hydrated—which is a challenge when exercising, especially in the heat. During exercise humans sweat and that water needs to be replaced!

How do you know how much water has been lost due to sweating? It is recommended that exercisers weigh themselves before and after exercise. Since a pint of water weighs about one pound, the water loss can be estimated by multiplying the weight lost by 1 pint. Losing four pounds during exercise would equal four pints or one-half gallon of water. This is not an unusual amount when exercising in the heat!

It is important to keep the body well hydrated at all times. By weighing yourself before and after exercise you can estimate how much water was lost and consciously plan to replace it by drinking more fluids.

4.2: Exercise Test Selection

In each of the testing categories that follow, the options for testing will be discussed. In general, there are no perfect exercise tests. The best tests are very accurate and very expensive. Realistically, everyone cannot have access to the best tests. Therefore, finding a test that is doable and provides useful information is the goal.

When selecting an exercise test the following should be considered: fitness goals, equipment, cost, accuracy, and skill. Based on the exercise goals identified, tests for each component of health-related fitness should be completed. Obviously the only test options are those for which there is testing equipment available. Additionally, the cost of the test must be considered. Many of the best tests may be cost prohibitive. The accuracy of the test is a major consideration. Ideally, the more accurate a test is the better. However, the test selection must be realistic. Consider the NFL combine. Here, potential

NFL players complete a series of exercise tests and their performance on these exercise tests can determine the draft order and potentially millions of dollars in future contracts. These tests must be very accurate and fair! On the other hand, recreational exercisers can get much benefit from exercise testing with less accuracy. The key is finding the test with the most accuracy that is realistically available. Finally, the better tests require skilled testers. For the following discussion several options will be presented along with simple exercise tests that can meet the SMART goals needs of recreational exercisers who want to maintain and improve health.

4.3: Cardiorespiratory Fitness Testing

The purpose of a cardiorespiratory fitness test is to determine the body's ability to take oxygen from the air in the environment and deliver to it the working cells during exercise. At maximal exercise, by pushing the body as hard as it can be pushed, the amount of oxygen used by the body is called the VO_2max. The VO_2max is one of the best indicators of health. The higher the VO_2max, the more oxygen that can be used and the better the body's organs are functioning.

The best way to measure the VO_2max is to complete a graded exercise test, generally on a treadmill, using a metabolic cart. This is an expensive, sophisticated test which is

MYTH BOX: THE HIGHER THE VO_2MAX THE FASTER THE DISTANCE RUNNING TIMES.

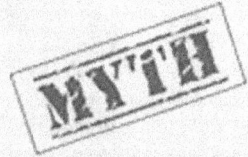

A really high VO_2max is definitely a great thing. Higher VO_2maxes are associated with many health benefits. A high VO_2max is also important for people who want to compete in long-distance events like marathons and triathlons. However, having the highest VO_2max does not always equate to winning these competitions. In fact, one of the most important qualities a long-distance endurance athlete can possess is a high anaerobic threshold.

The anaerobic threshold represents the point at which athletes "switch" from primarily relying on aerobic metabolism to meet energy demands to primarily anaerobic metabolism. When exercise is not very intense, like walking, we rely mainly on aerobic metabolism to meet energy needs. As exercise becomes more intense, aerobic metabolism cannot make the small molecules needed for energy fast enough to continue exercising at that intensity. At this point, anaerobic metabolism ramps up. The chemical reactions in anaerobic metabolism occur more quickly than during aerobic metabolism. However, there is a consequence of anaerobic metabolism and this is the production of lactic acid. Lactic acid plays havoc on muscular contractions and quickly causes fatigue.

In long-distance races, having a higher anaerobic threshold means being able to run faster without producing too much lactic acid. Consider the following example:

Brailey has a VO_2max of 60 ml/kg/min and Elliana has a VO_2max of 50 ml/kg/min. Brailey, however, has an anaerobic threshold that occurs when she runs faster than 5mph. Elliana's doesn't happen until she runs faster than 5.1mph. This would mean that Elliana, though having a lower VO_2max, could run a race faster than Brailey.

In order to improve anaerobic threshold, long-distance endurance athletes need to spend time exercising at or above intensities that produce lactic acid. Doing so will delay the anaerobic threshold and permit the athlete to run, cycle, or swim at higher speeds before accumulating too much lactic acid. However, athletes also cannot neglect long-distance training days. It is surely a balancing act.

not available to most people. For example, the exerciser would run on a treadmill while hooked up to a metabolic cart. All of the air expired by the exerciser is collected through a tube and analyzed by the computer in the cart. The amount of oxygen burned by the body is reported in milliliters.

Since most students will not have the option of a full-blown graded exercise test, other tests are available to estimate VO_2max. These can also be higher cost and require the services of a trained tester. Options might include a treadmill, bicycle, or step test without the metabolic cart, or various run tests.

Students who want to determine their starting point or track changes over time in cardiorespiratory fitness can administer their own test or test each other with a group of friends. A good test for beginners is the 12-minute walk/run test. By using a local track with a known distance, the exerciser can run or walk as fast as possible for 12 minutes. The distance covered is recorded. This test can be administered periodically (such as every 3 or 6 months) to see the changes made by the training program.

YOUR TURN 4.1

Cardiorespiratory Test

12-Minute Run/Walk

Directions: Find a running track with a known distance. Most outdoor tracks are one-quarter mile on the inside lane. Indoor tracks are generally shorter. Set your watch timer to 12 minutes. Start the timer and begin to run or walk as fast as you can, pacing yourself knowing that you have to continue for 12 minutes. Make sure to count the number of laps. When 12 minutes has expired note where you are on the track. You may have to estimate the distance completed on the final lap. Make sure you record your distance and keep it in a safe place where you can access it at a later date.

Date_____ Distance completed in 12 minutes _____ yards

[1/4 mile = 440 yards]
If using a ¼ mile track: Yards completed = Laps completed × 440 + fraction of last lap × 440

4.4: Muscular Strength Testing

As previously mentioned, the ability of muscles to generate force is called strength. Making an assessment of overall strength is challenging because there are many muscles in the body and the ability to generate muscular force is different at each of the joints. Even the same muscles on the right and left sides likely have different measures for strength. Therefore, when testing for strength the tests should consider muscle groups that are commonly used in day-to-day activities.

The best tests for evaluating muscular strength use expensive equipment called isokinetic machines. These are electronic devices that regulate the movement speed and record the amount of force being generated. They can be set up to evaluate the strength of almost any joint, left and right sides separately. They are primarily used in rehab settings to evaluate the strength of injured joints.

Another way to test muscular strength is to use devices called dynamometers. There are different types of dynamometers for different joints of the body. There is little movement in the dynamometer but it displays the pounds of force generated. The test has a limited range of movement, but it does give a very measurable quantity of force generation.

A more commonly used strength test is the one-rep maximum. This test involves finding the maximum weight the exerciser can lift one time. However, this is not simple to do for the first time. The amount of weight to begin with is so variable among people that it is difficult to determine. If too little weight is chosen, the weight must be increased. Similarly, if too much weight is chosen, the weight must be decreased. By making an inaccurate estimate, the exerciser will have to lift weights more times and fatigue will set in. If there is fatigue, then the true one-rep max may be underrepresented. Fortunately, when follow-up testing is done at a later date, the data from the previous test can be used to determine a good starting weight.

A simpler test is to use a set weight and count the number of times it is lifted before fatigue. Because it involves more than one rep during the test, it is not the best. Lifting multiple times without rest is more like muscular endurance but can still provide evidence of improving strength. In some situations, this test might be the best option. When testing for strength, it is better to use an exercise that involves several joints as opposed to one joint. For example, the bench press uses the shoulder, elbow, and wrist joints, while the squat uses the hip, knee, and ankle joints. A good choice is the bench press. Males would use 150 pounds and females 100 pounds. The weight should be set on the bar or machine and the number of reps counted and recorded. Over time an effective resistance training program would result in more reps being completed. Due to variations in equipment, it is important to use the same machines or free weights when doing follow-up testing!

YOUR TURN 4.2

Muscle Strength Test
Bench Press Test

Directions: Go to a fitness facility and find a bench press machine. Free weights can also be used but be sure to have a spotter with you. Males should use 150 pounds and females 100 pounds. The weight should be set on the bar or machine. Count the number of reps completed to exhaustion. Record the number of reps completed.

Date_____

Number of bench press reps completed _____

Remember this is not the best test for measuring true muscular strength. However, it will measure strength to some degree and is manageable for a self-test. Improvements in strength will be obvious if you keep a log of lifting workouts and notice the increases in weight lifted on a weekly basis.

4.5: Muscular Endurance Testing

The ability to contract a muscle repeatedly is muscular endurance. Testing for muscular endurance is one of the simpler components of fitness to measure. Like strength testing it is good to use exercises that involve multiple joints or the muscles of the trunk. Classic tests for muscular endurance include curl-ups and push-ups. Like any tests, proper technique must be used. The exerciser repeats the exercise until fatigued. Some tests use a cadence of a certain number of reps per minute (e.g., 20 per minute or one every 3 seconds). Other tests do not use a cadence and the exercisers do the test at their own pace.

For the push-up test, males begin on their hands and toes. Females can begin the same as males or on their hands and knees. When the test begins the exerciser completes as many reps as possible using proper form. The number of reps is counted and recorded.

For the curl-up test, the exerciser should lie flat on the back with knees bent and arms crossed over the chest. Each curl-up rep requires movement at the abdomen and the shoulder blades should move off the ground before returning. The exerciser should use proper form while counting and recording the total number of reps.

Other tests for muscular endurance include pull-ups, planks, and body squats. Pull-ups involve the number of times the body can be lifted while hanging from a bar by bending the elbows and shoulders, while body squats involve the number of times a person can bend at the knees and hips from a standing position and return. Planks are measured in time that a person can hold a straight back while resting on the forearms and toes.

Muscle Endurance Tests

Push-Up Test

Directions: Find a space that is large enough to do a push-up comfortably. Place a rolled towel under the chest. Keeping the back straight, support your body on your hands and toes. Females can choose to support the body on the hands and knees. Lower the body by bending the elbows until your chest touches the towel. Then return to the starting position. Repeat until the arms fatigue and/or proper form (straight back) cannot be maintained. Record the number of push-ups completed.

Curl-Up Test

Directions: Find a space that is large enough to lie flat on your back comfortably. Bend your knees 45 degrees with your feet flat on the floor. Cross your arms over your chest. When ready slowly curl up at the waist bringing your shoulder blades off the floor and slowly return. Repeat until the abdominal muscles fatigue and/or proper form cannot be maintained. Record the number of curl-ups completed.

Date_____

Number of push-ups completed _____

Number of curl-ups completed _____

4.6: Flexibility Testing

Like muscular strength and muscular endurance, an individual's flexibility varies at different joints. The more a joint can be moved through its full range of motion the more flexibility there is at the joint. Professionals will often use a goniometer to measure the degrees of the range of motion for a joint. Measuring many joints takes time and requires skill. Therefore, the sit-and-reach is often used to measure general flexibility. The exerciser sits with the feet (shoes off) against a sit-and-reach bench. With the legs straight the person being tested reaches as far forward as possible and a measurement is taken in inches of the distance below or above the bottom of the foot.

This test can be modified for those who do not have access to a sit-and-reach bench. All that is required is a step and a ruler. The exerciser can stand on a bench or step and bend over with the knees straight. A partner can measure the distance the fingertips go past the bottom of the foot (or above the bottom of the foot). For consistency it is important that the exerciser does not wear shoes and moves toward the foot in a slow and controlled fashion.

YOUR TURN 4.4

Flexibility Test

Trunk Flexion Test

Directions: Get a partner to help with this test. Find a ruler and a stair step or a bench that can support your weight. Remove your shoes. With your toes on the end of the bench or step bend at the waist and reach as far as you can toward or past your toes with your knees straight and one hand on top of the other. Move in a controlled fashion without bouncing. Have your partner measure the distance between your fingertips and top of the bench or step in inches. If you cannot reach to the bench record a negative number in inches. If you reach past the bottom of the bench record a positive number in inches. Repeat three times. Record the highest number representing your best trial.

Date_____

Trial 1 + / - _____ inches

Trial 2 + / - _____ inches

Trial 3 + / - _____ inches

Best Trial + / - _____ inches

4.7: Neuromotor Testing

A recent fitness testing area to get attention is neuromotor. This type of testing often assesses balance. Balance testing is a little tricky and requires skill to do it correctly. There are various tests that include standing in different positions or jumping in different patterns. A simple test to get an idea of balance is to see how long the exerciser can stand on the non-dominate foot with the eyes closed without putting the other foot down.

YOUR TURN 4.5

Neuromotor Test

Balance Test

Directions: Find a place with enough room to allow for five feet of empty space around you. Have a partner keep the time. Remove your shoes. Begin by standing on your <u>non-dominate</u> leg with your eyes closed and hands on your hips. On command start timing and determine how long you can balance in that position without taking your hands off your hips, opening your eyes, or putting your other foot on the floor. Record the time the balance position was held.

Date_____

Time _____ seconds

4.8: Body Composition Testing

The human body primarily comprises muscle, fat, water, and minerals. While the body needs a minimum amount of all of these components for good health, too much fat is unhealthy. When assessing body composition, the focus tends to be on the amount of fat. From a health standpoint the percent of the body that is made up of fat is an important value. Males should have 10 to 15 percent body fat and women should have 15 to 20 percent.

There are many tests to determine or estimate percent body fat. Some are very clinical and require sophisticated equipment. The original method was underwater (or hydrostatic) weighing. This is a tedious test where an individual's body density is determined by comparing the body weight in air with the body weight when submerged in water. The basic concept is fat floats, which means the body is less dense. People with more body fat will weigh less in the water than people with less body fat. Using underwater weighing as a reference, many techniques using skinfold calipers were developed. The common method measures the thickness of fat beneath the skin on various sites on the body. With a skilled tester, skinfolds are an excellent way to measure body fat. Also, from underwater weighing other techniques using electronic instruments were developed such as bioelectrical impedance and near-infrared spectroscopy. These methods can be accurate as well if they are done properly.

A simple calculation to evaluate body composition uses height and weight. The Body Mass Index (BMI) is a person's weight in kilograms divided by a person's height in meters squared. Since there is no direct or indirect measure of body fat, this method does not discriminate between the different components that make up the person's weight. It is simply a measure of the weight in relation to height. Therefore, it is not the most informative measure of body composition. Despite this it is widely used because it is relatively easy to compute. BMI is the most common of all the methods. A quick calculation provides a value indicating whether a person's weight is considered healthy (18.5 to 24.9). Under 18.5 is indicative of underweight and 25 to 29.9 is overweight. A score of 30 or above would be classified as obese. One major limitation of this method is that individuals with large muscles could be classified as overweight or obese when in fact they possess a healthy amount of fat.

YOUR TURN 4.6

Body Composition Test
BMI Test

Directions: Determine your height in inches and your weight in pounds.

Date_____

Height_____(inches)   Weight_____(pounds)

Convert both to metric:

Height _____ inches × .0254 = _____ meters

Weight _____ pounds / 2.2 = _____ kilograms

Square the height:

Height _____ meters × Height _____ meters = _____ meters^2

Calculate BMI:

Weight _____ kilograms / Height^2 _____Meters^2 = _____kilograms/
meters^2

Compare with recommended values:

Underweight <18.5

Normal   18.5–24.9

Overweight   25.0–29.9

Obese >30.0

4.9: Exercise Testing Session and Order

For exercise testing results to be meaningful, the tests must be conducted the same way every time and in a logical order. Ideally the tests should be done using the same equipment by the same tester on the same indoor surfaces. Unfortunately, this is seldom possible but it should be done when feasible. Any variations in testing will affect the results and make comparisons from one test session to the next less accurate.

All testing sessions must include a warm-up to prepare the body for physical activity. The warm-up will be discussed in detail in the next section.

Once the body is warmed up the physical testing can begin. The order in which the tests are performed is very important. Non-physical tests such as height, weight, and other body composition tests should be done first and can actually be done before the warm-up. Then after the warm-up, tests that involve skill should be done first. Skill tests are not as big of a factor in exercise testing for health as compared with the testing of athletes. Of those discussed, neuromotor testing would come first since balance requires some skill. After the skill tests the order would follow with the least intense tests to those that are most intense because exercisers do not want to be totally fatigued early in the session. Attention should also be paid to the size of the muscle groups being used in the test. Larger muscle groups should be tested before the smaller muscle groups. For example, the shoulder muscles should be tested before the elbow muscles.

With these objectives in mind, after the body composition tests the warm-up should be done. Then the skills tests can be followed by flexibility which is low intensity. Moving on, the next tests would be muscular strength starting with the largest muscle groups to the smallest (if multiple strength tests are done). Next would be the muscular endurance tests followed by cardiorespiratory tests. It is not necessary to do all of the testing in one day, and it is often good to break the session into more than one to avoid fatiguing the exercisers over one long session in one day.

YOUR TURN 4.7

Exercise Testing Order

Directions: Choose a test for each of the following:

Muscular Endurance _____

Muscular Strength _____

Flexibility _____

Cardiorespiratory Fitness _____

Body Composition _____

Neuromotor Fitness _____

If you were going to test all of the above in one day, list the order of testing:

1. _____

2. _____

3. _____

4. _____

5. _____

6. _____

4.10: Components of an Exercise Training Session

A well-designed exercise program should include four components in each training session: warm-up, conditioning, cool-down, and stretching. Conditioning is the longest and most detailed part of the four and will be discussed in detail in the next section. Although shorter in duration, the warm-up and cool-down are still very important and stretching is highly recommended.

The purpose of the warm-up is to prepare the body for intense exercise. This is accomplished by 5 to 10 minutes of light activity such as jogging and light stretching. The first objective is to gradually increase the body's temperature. When the body temperature increases a few degrees, the efficiency of the body functions will improve. Muscles will contract better and more blood will flow to the parts of the body that need it most. Stretching will loosen the muscles to allow them to move more freely. All together the warm-up can help to improve performance during exercise to get a better workout and potentially decrease the chance of injury. Breaking into a light sweat is a sign that the body is warmed up.

The cool-down is needed to gradually prepare the body for rest. During exercise most of the body's functions such as heart rate, breathing, and burning calories are significantly elevated. It is best for the body to gradually lower these functions instead of slowing them down abruptly. This is easily accomplished by 5 to 10 minutes of light activity such as walking briskly and gradually slowing the pace. A guide to know when the body has cooled down is a heart rate of under 100 beats per minute. Following the light activity is a good time to do stretching exercises to improve flexibility. The guidelines for developing flexibility are presented in the next section and should be included as part of each training session.

4.11: Guidelines for Conditioning

When designing the conditioning portion of the exercise program professionals follow the FITT-VP principle developed by the American College of Sports Medicine.[1] FITT-VP is an acronym for frequency, intensity, time, type, volume, and progression. The type of exercise to be done is determined by considering the SMART goals that were developed. Then the frequency (or number of times per week) of exercise needs to be decided along with how long (time) and how hard (intensity) to exercise during each session. How much total exercise (volume) and how fast to increase the volume (progression) are also considered.

The FITT-VP principle can be applied to each of the components of fitness discussed, with the exception of body composition. The major components of cardiorespiratory fitness, strength, and flexibility will be discussed in detail.

VOICES FROM CAMPUS 4.1

LaTonya

When I was in high school I ran track and focused on short-distance sprinting. I could have run track at several Division III schools but none had my major and I decided to attend a large, state university. I knew without track I needed to start an exercise program. When I went to orientation I learned that the rec center had a lot of exercise options and trainers who could help me get started. So when I got to school I went to talk with a trainer.

I was surprised when I starting talking with the trainer that the exercises I had been doing all my life were not the best exercises for health. She said that exercise is specific and different goals require very different programs. Who would have thought that running sprints and lifting heavier weights a few reps per set was not the best program for my long-term health!

My trainer told me about the FITT-VP principle and designed a program for the "new me." Now I am running longer distances and lifting lighter weight more times per set. This has been a real adjustment but I am slowly adjusting. Fortunately, my trainer started me slowly and gradually increased my distances and weights. I am not able to sprint as fast as when I was in high school but I do feel healthier. I think I can do this for the rest of my life!

Cardiorespiratory Fitness

The type of exercises that will improve cardiorespiratory fitness are generally known as aerobic exercises. They are typically vigorous, continuous, and rhythmic exercises and include activities such as walking, jogging, running, cycling, swimming, rowing, and cross-country skiing. These activities all have repeating movements that can be done continuously. Also included are sports that are not as rhythmic (e.g., soccer, basketball, racket sports, downhill skiing, and hiking). These less rhythmical activities should only be done by individuals who have at least an average level of fitness. In other words, beginners should focus on rhythmic activities that they are able to perform continuously.

The intensity of aerobic exercises will depend on the individual's desire to exercise moderately or vigorously. For example, moderate exercise would be performed at a walking pace and vigorous exercise would be performed at a jogging/running pace. For vigorous exercise, individuals would want to work at 70 percent to 85 percent of their maximum heart rate. It is easy to estimate maximum heart rate by subtracting the person's age from 220. This formula works well with healthy individuals but should be avoided by people with certain diseases or those who are taking medications that affect heart rate. A 20-year-old student would have an estimated maximum heart rate of 220 - 20 = 200 beats per minute (bpm). By multiplying 200 by .70

and .85, a target zone of 170 bpm to 190 bpm is determined. This means that this student would want to exercise for the designated time between 170 bpm and 190 bpm. These heart rates can be observed by using a heart rate monitor or taking a pulse (such as at the wrist) periodically during the exercise session. If the pulse rate drops below 170 bpm, then the student needs to increase the intensity by moving faster. If the pulse rate increases above 190 bpm, the student needs to slow down the pace. By doing this the student will be able to exercise safely while getting the maximum benefit from the workout. If the student chooses to do moderate exercise, it is still good to take periodic heart rates. Walkers should walk at a range of 50 percent to 70 percent of maximum heart rate (100 bpm to 140 bpm for a 20-year-old [200 × .5 = 100, 200 × .7 = 140]).

The frequency of exercise will depend on the intensity of exercise. The basic recommendation is at least three times per week for vigorous exercisers and at least five times per week for moderate exercisers. While increasing these frequencies per week will provide more health benefits it is important to remember that the human body does need rest and recovery. Therefore, more is better only to a point; it is possible to do too much. Vigorous exercisers should do cardiovascular workouts three to five times per week while moderate exercisers should do cardiovascular workouts five to seven times per week. These ranges should be determined with consideration to the number of other workouts done per week, particularly strength training.

The recommended time (duration) of the conditioning portion of the workout is 30 to 60 minutes per day for moderate intensities and 20 to 60 minutes per day for vigorous intensities. These are fairly wide ranges so a good target would be 45 minutes for moderate exercisers and 30 to 40 minutes for vigorous exercisers. For exercisers who are deconditioned, it is acceptable to alternate walking and running during the workout. For example, if a student wants to begin running and cannot run for 20 minutes, the student could run for 10 minutes, walk for 5 minutes, and then run for 10 more minutes. Gradually over time the student can increase the time running until reaching the 20-minute goal of continuous running. Then the student can add minutes every week until being able to run for 40 or more minutes without stopping or walking.

The volume portion of the FITT-VP sets goals for how much total work will be done per week. It is a combination of intensity, frequency, and time (duration). There are several ways to measure volume but some would require the help of a fitness trainer. The easiest way is to use a step counter with a goal of 7,000 steps per day, assuming the equipment is available. If measurements of volume are not reasonable to make, then focusing on the other FITT-VP principles can still be effective.

The concept of overload was discussed in Chapter 3. In order to continue to make improvements in health and fitness the workouts must continue to get harder. This is the progression principle of the FITT-VP. Doing the same workout continuously will lead to stagnation and a tapering off of improvements. In the cardiorespiratory area this means that increasing the intensity, time (duration), and/or frequency gradually over the months or year is required. The benefits of periodic fitness testing in this circumstance are obvious. Improvements, if they are there, will be evident from the tests and the test results can be used to decide whether the exercise program needs to be redesigned. Then the intensity (heart rate targets), number of workouts per week, or duration of exercise per session can be increased to stimulate continuous improvements.

YOUR TURN 4.8

Cardiorespiratory Program Design

Directions: List two SMART goals for your cardiorespiratory fitness. (Refer to Your Turn 3.1. You may already have them!) Then develop a cardiorespiratory fitness program using the FITT-VP principle.

SMART Goal 1: _____

_____

SMART Goal 2: _____

_____

Frequency of Exercise: _____times/week

Intensity of Exercise: _____bpm to _____bpm

Type of Exercise: _____

Time of Exercise: _____minutes

*Not sure what type of aerobic exercise you may want to do? Do an Internet search for these keywords: cardiorespiratory fitness exercise examples or cardiovascular fitness exercise examples. Go to a fitness center and see what types of equipment are available. Talk with your friends who exercise about activities they like to do.

Resistance Training for Strength Improvements

The FITT-VP principle can also be used for developing resistance training programs. The variables that need to be determined include the number of exercises, sets, reps, and the rest time between exercises. Sets are the number of times each exercise is repeated in one workout. A typical range is between one and four sets. The number of times a lift is done in each set is the reps or repetitions. A typical range for reps is between 8 and 20.

To improve strength the type of exercises required are those that stress the muscles by applying resistance. The resistance used to increase strength can be free weights, weight machines, hydraulic machines, isokinetic machines, or virtually anything that resists muscle contractions. There is continuous debate about which type of resistance or equipment is best. In reality for individuals who want to improve health any form of resistance will work. The debate over which is best should be left to trainers of elite athletes. Only athletes competing at the higher levels stand to benefit more from the specific resistance training equipment used. Exercisers for health should use what equipment is available and put forth a good effort to overload the muscles. The result will be an improvement in strength.

The intensity of lifting is determined by a percent of the maximum weight a person can lift with any specific exercise. This is called the one-rep maximum or 1RM. Determining a 1RM is a little tricky and it is beneficial to work with a trainer to find these quicker. However, with trial and error the 1RM weights can be determined over a few workouts. In general beginners should use 40 percent to 50 percent of their 1RM. Those with limited experience can advance to 60 percent to 70 percent of 1RM. Experienced lifters can use 80 percent or more of the 1RM. Of course these intensities must be considered with the other FITT-VP principles to get the actual percents when designing the complete workout plan.

Using the trial-and-error approach to determine initial lifting weight intensities begins with determining the other variables, including the number of sets and reps. After deciding on the target number of reps (which will be discussed later in this chapter) the lifter will start with a light weight and see how many reps can be completed. If the number completed is more than the target, the weight will be increased for the next set. If unable to attain the target reps, the weight will be decreased for the next set. This is repeated until the target reps are reached within one rep of the goal for the set.

The recommended frequency or number of times lifting per week is two to three. Strength can be maintained by lifting once per week, but if a week is missed strength begins to decline. Therefore, two is the recommended minimum. Lifting should be a maximal workout which results in major fatigue of the muscles. Consequently, the muscles worked need time to recover and should not be used for lifting the following day. It is generally recommended to allow at least one day off after a resistance workout resulting in a maximum recommendation of three workouts per week. It is acceptable to lift more than three times per week if all muscles are not worked in the same session. If, for example, the shoulders and arms are worked one day, the legs the second day, and the trunk the third day, it would be possible to lift six days per week. This is tolerable because one muscle group gets two days of rest while the other muscle groups are being worked on different days. However, this is more lifting than is necessary to maintain good health. This high-frequency program would be more appropriate for athletes preparing for competition.

The time spent on resistance training varies widely and specific guidelines are not established. The time will depend on the number of exercises, the number of sets, the number of reps, and the time of rest between exercises. Considering all of these variables it would be good to keep the conditioning time of the program between 30 and 40 minutes. This provides time for warm-up, cool-down, and stretching.

As previously mentioned, an important consideration in resistance training design is the number of repetitions planned per set. There have been many studies on the ideal number of reps. The general guideline is 8 to 12 to get improvements in strength. If the goal is more muscular endurance, then the reps should be increased to 15 to 20. Since many young exercisers are interested in appearance as well as health, using higher weights and doing about eight reps would be recommended. This amount will cause more muscle growth than doing higher reps. However, as health becomes the objective, higher reps with lower weights should be attempted.

The recommended number of sets to improve strength is two to four. However, one set has been shown to be effective for less-experienced lifters and those focusing on muscular endurance. From a health standpoint it is more important that lifting be done regularly than trying to get higher numbers of sets. An important factor with this issue is time. A one-set workout takes much less time than a three-set workout!

As previously mentioned resistance training should be a maximal workout and recovery time is absolutely needed. Therefore, rest and recovery must be considered in the overall workout design. First, any muscle groups worked in a resistance training session need a day off and should not be trained again for 48 hours. Recovery is also needed during a workout between each set. Two to three minutes is generally recommended. These recovery times must be considered in the program design in relation to how long a session will be and how many sessions will be completed per week.

The final FITT-VP principles are volume and progression. The volume of resistance training can be computed by totaling all of the weight lifted per week. This would be the frequency times weight times sets times reps. While it may not be necessary to compute this number, it does provide a value for the amount of work done and could be useful to quantify when the lifter is overtraining. There is no recommended volume guideline. However, progression is an important principle.

Without continuing to overload the body's systems improvement will not be made. This can be very obvious in resistance training. For example, after bench pressing 200 pounds, eight reps, for two sets, twice per week it will become easier. To continue to gain strength the lifter must increase at least one of the variables. The weight could be increased to 210 pounds. The reps could be increased to 10 reps. Two sets could be increased to three. Or the frequency could be increased to three times per week. The typical variable to increase is the weight. A good guideline is when the target reps (eight in the above example) are exceeded by two reps in two consecutive workouts, then 5 percent to 10 percent should be added to the weight. Therefore, instead of lifting 200 pounds the weight would be increased to 210 pounds. (Generally 5 percent is used for the arms and 10 percent is used for the legs and trunk.)

YOUR TURN 4.9

Resistance Training Program Design

Directions: List two SMART goals for your muscular strength and endurance fitness. (Refer to Your Turn 3.1. You may already have them!). Then develop a resistance training program using the FITT-VP principle.

SMART Goal 1: _____

_____

SMART Goal 2: _____

_____

Frequency of Exercise: _____times/week

Intensity of Exercise: _____ percent of 1RM

Type of Exercise (list 8–10 resistance training exercises):

1. _____

2. _____

3. _____

4. _____

5. _____

6. _____

7. _____

8. _____

9. _____

10. _____

Repetitions per set _____reps/set Sets per workout _____sets/workout

*Not sure what resistance training exercises you may want to do? Do an Internet search for these keywords: resistance training exercises, resistance

training exercise videos, weight training exercises, or weight training exercise videos. Go to a fitness center and see what types of equipment are available. Talk with your friends who do resistance training about exercises they like to do. Remember to select exercises that work a variety of muscle groups, and most should have movements at more than one joint.

Flexibility Training

Training flexibility is different from cardiorespiratory and resistance because there is much less fatigue. Still, the FITT-VP principle can be used. In Chapter 2 the different types of stretching were discussed. While all can be effective, it is recommended to focus on static stretching. Slowly stretching the target muscle group to the point of slight discomfort and holding it from 10 to 60 seconds is recommended. Static stretching is the safest and can be done alone. A program of approximately 10 exercises that include the major muscle groups is sufficient.

The frequency of the stretching workout should be at least two to three times per week. However, more frequently or even daily is more effective. Since stretching does not require much recovery time it can be performed more often. It should be done when the muscles are warm. Following the cool-down of the cardiorespiratory or resistance workout is an ideal time.

The intensity of the stretch is quite easy to monitor. As the stretch progresses, the muscles begin to feel tighter. When there is a slight feeling of discomfort the muscle is well stretched and the position should be held.

The time to hold the stretch at the point of slight discomfort should be 10 to 30 seconds. The actual time will depend on the number of times the stretch will be completed. The best way to determine the number of stretches and the hold times is to consider the volume. Generally, each stretch should be held for a total of 60 seconds. Therefore, the stretch can be done two times for 30 seconds, six times for 10 seconds, or any combination in between.

In order to continue to make improvements or progress the stretches must always be to the point of slight discomfort. Over time the stretch will become greater to get to that discomfort point. Additionally, it is not necessary to continually improve flexibility. Once good flexibility is attained it is only necessary to maintain it. Maintenance can be accomplished by continuing to stretch regularly to point of slight discomfort.

YOUR TURN 4.10

Flexibility Program Design

Directions: List two SMART goals for your flexibility fitness. (Refer to Your Turn 3.1. You may already have them!). Then develop a flexibility program using the FITT-VP principle.

SMART Goal 1: _____

_____

SMART Goal 2: _____

_____

Frequency of Exercise: _____times/week

Intensity of Exercise: _____

Type of Exercise (list 8–10 flexibility exercises):

1. _____

2. _____

3. _____

4. _____

5. _____

6. _____

7. _____

8. _____

9. _____

10. _____

Time of Exercise: Hold each stretch _____seconds and repeat _____ times per session

*Not sure what type of flexibility exercise you may want to do? Do an Internet search for these keywords: flexibility exercises or flexibility exercise examples. Talk with your friends who exercise about stretches they like to do. Consider a variety of exercises that include all major joints of the body.

Neuromotor Training

Neuromotor training has not been studied as much as cardiorespiratory, resistance, and flexibility training and therefore less is known about it. The benefits appear to be greater in older individuals. Nevertheless, college-aged students may enjoy and benefit from neuromotor training. Some types of neuromotor training include yoga and Tai Chi. Some of these will be described in Chapter 6. It is recommended to participate in these types of activities two to three times per week for 20 to 30 minutes. Of course these activities take time. It is recommended that young people participate in neuromotor activities only after the minimum of three cardiorespiratory and two resistance workouts per week.

4.12: Periodization

Maintaining an exercise program for life requires strategies to keep exercise fun and energizing. Professional trainers use periodization to keep their athletes engaged and from being overtrained. Periodization was developed in the Soviet Union in the 1960s for professional and Olympic weight lifters. It has been modified over the years for use with many different types of athletes. The principles can be used by all exercisers.

Periodization is a process of planning exercise programs for the long term by varying the intensity and volume of work to avoid overtraining and injuries. Lessons from periodization that can be used by mainstream exercisers include changing the exercise program periodically to bring in new activities and work the body and muscles in new ways. By changing the exercise program, it will not become too routine and the exercisers will be more likely to continue with it and improve their health.

4.13: The Take Away

- It is important to keep an exercise log and monitor exercise program progress with periodic fitness testing.

- Exercise tests should align with exercise goals and include, at the minimum, cardiorespiratory, strength, and flexibility tests.

- The exercise session should include warm-up, conditioning, and cool-down. Flexibility training should be added to most sessions.

- Conditioning design should consider the FITT-VP principle: frequency, intensity, time, type, volume, and progression.

- The long-term exercise plan should consider periodization, varying volume and intensity throughout the year to avoid over-training and staleness.

References

1. American College of Sports Medicine. (2018). *ACSM's guidelines for exercise testing and prescription* (10th ed.). Philadelphia, PA: Wolters Kluwer Health.

COMPLEMENTING AN EXERCISE PROGRAM WITH PHYSICAL ACTIVITY

Okay, I have designed my exercise program. Why do I need to do other activities?

A t this point, this book has presented numerous topics. From the health-related consequences of physical inactivity to exercise program design, this book has sought to equip readers with the best knowledge for identifying their needs for regular exercise, establishing exercise goals, and designing an individualized exercise program for addressing individual needs and goals. Now this book will move to the "lighter" side of exercise program design and discuss complementing an exercise program with other forms of physical activity.

Having an exercise program in place and actually adhering to that program is a fantastic achievement. Risks for disease will be reduced, attentiveness will be enhanced, and everyday productivity and well-being will be improved as a result of this adherence. However, to maximize the effectiveness of an exercise program and really drive down chronic disease risk, exercise alone may not be enough. There is no doubt that adhering to an exercise program is a phenomenal accomplishment and will certainly improve a person's health by leaps and bounds! However, there is still a need for further physical activity beyond an exercise program as too much "downtime" between exercise sessions can actually be detrimental to overall health. This chapter will focus on identifying the risks associated with prolonged sitting and sedentary times and methods for overcoming these risks. Furthermore, attention will be paid to identifying useful forms of physical activity that can be built into the structure of everyday routines.

5.1: Sedentary Behaviors and Health

Most adults are well aware of the negative consequences associated with inactivity. In fact, this book has discussed those very consequences. However, in this book, there has yet to be a distinction made between physical inactivity and sedentary behaviors. Physical inactivity is often defined as failing to perform moderate intensity physical activity.[6] Moderate intensity was discussed in Chapter 4. Activities like brisk walks, mowing the lawn, playing a pickup game of basketball, or playing backyard tag football would be considered moderate intensity physical activities. Sedentary behaviors, on the other hand, are actually different from basic physical inactivity. Sedentary behaviors are those behaviors and activities that burn less than 1.5 times the calories required to simply maintain life.[6] Therefore, activities that only increase caloric expenditures 0.5 times the amount needed to stay alive do not require much effort at all. Much to the disappointment of public health officials, increasingly too many people engage in too many sedentary behaviors and these behaviors are very bad for overall health.

Physiological necessities like breathing, regulating body temperature, and maintaining a heartbeat all require the burning of calories. At rest, this caloric expenditure is referred to as the basal metabolic rate. The basal metabolic rate represents the caloric expenditure required for just staying alive. Activities that only increase the caloric expenditure by a mere 0.5 times this basic requirement are considered sedentary activities. Examples of these activities include your basic couch potato behaviors. Activities like sitting in a recliner and watching television, lounging on the couch and playing video games, and even sitting behind a desk and writing an exercise book are all activities that would be classified as sedentary behaviors. These sedentary behaviors can actually prove to be more devastating for overall health than physical inactivity. What is more, engaging in sedentary behaviors for lengthy periods of time can "wash out" many of the benefits of adhering to a well-designed exercise program! Therefore, even though people exercise regularly, they must continue to stay in motion and avoid excessive sedentary behaviors.

Several studies in recent years have sought to examine the impact of sedentary behaviors on health, disease, and mortality risk. Prolonged periods of engaging in sedentary behaviors, like being a couch potato or sitting behind a desk at work, have been associated with a variety of adverse health consequences. First, prolonged engagement in sedentary behaviors appears to lead to increases in abdominal fat, fats in the blood, and insulin levels.[4] The increase in insulin levels represents a state of insulin resistance, meaning it is more likely that blood glucose levels will rise as well. Furthermore, prolonged sedentary behavior causes the level of good cholesterol (HDL) in the blood to plummet.[4] These adverse consequences combine to form what is known as metabolic syndrome. Metabolic syndrome consists of having three of the following five risk factors for cardiovascular disease: high blood pressure, high triglycerides (fats in the blood), high abdominal fat, elevated blood glucose, and low HDL. Having metabolic syndrome puts people on the fast track to cardiovascular disease and type 2 diabetes. Overall, sedentary time is associated with increased risks of developing type 2 diabetes, cardiovascular disease, and all-cause mortality.[10] Shockingly, prolonged sedentary time is still predictive of negative health outcomes, even if someone is still physically active![1] The message is clear: exercise must be complemented with more physical activity and reduced sedentary time!

YOUR TURN 5.1

Identifying Sedentary Behaviors

Directions: Now that you know the definition of a sedentary behavior and some examples of these behaviors, identify five sedentary behaviors that you engage in on a regular basis. Further, list how much time per day you spend doing each sedentary behavior. Lastly, state whether you believe these sedentary behaviors are detrimental to your overall health and explain why or why not.

Sedentary Behavior	How much time per day, or week if it is not a daily behavior, do you spend doing this activity (in minutes)?
1.	
2.	
3.	
4.	
5.	
Do you believe these sedentary behaviors are detrimental to YOUR health? Why or why not?	

Sitting Is the New Smoking

For many years, researchers and healthcare professionals were aware of the adverse consequences associated with prolonged sitting time. Too much time spent in a seated position is associated with numerous adverse health consequences. These consequences include increases in abdominal fat, body weight, blood pressure, fats in the blood, post-meal blood glucose levels, and insulin resistance.[7] Additionally, increased sitting time is linked to lower HDL. Therefore, prolonged sitting time, similar to prolonged sedentary behavior, is linked to metabolic syndrome. In sum, prolonged sitting time leads to increases in the risks for cardiovascular disease, cancer, type 2 diabetes, and all-cause death.[5, 7, 8]

It is known that prolonged sitting time is associated with many adverse health consequences. But the question is why? When someone sits, not only is that person expending fewer calories, but blood flow becomes restricted as well. The restriction in blood flow leads to a subsequent increase in what are known as clotting factors. These clotting factors lead to the production of blood clots and these blood clots can find themselves lodged in fat deposits in the arteries, leading to cardiac or pulmonary events. For the long term, the disruption in blood flow associated with sitting causes damage to the walls of arteries. This damage, coupled with expending fewer calories, really begins and accelerates the atherosclerosis cascade which will eventually lead to cardiovascular disease.

These disruptions in normal physiology ultimately account for the adverse health consequences previously discussed.

For years the decision to smoke cigarettes has been the worst decision one could make as it pertains to overall health. Today, that decision may be the second worst decision one could make! It is estimated that one hour of sitting can take 22 minutes off of a person's life expectancy. While for every cigarette smoked, 11 minutes come off a person's life expectancy.[9] Similar to sedentary behaviors, even if people adhere to a well-designed exercise program yet engage in prolonged sitting time, the benefits of exercise can be diminished. So if the goal of exercise is to improve health, regular exercise should be complemented with physical activities!

YOUR TURN 5.2

Sitting Time

Directions: Now that you know sitting for prolonged periods of time is detrimental to overall health, please calculate how many times in one day you sit for one consecutive hour. Based on the estimate that one consecutive hour of sitting equals a 22-minute reduction in life expectancy, calculate how many minutes you would lose off your expected life expectancy in one week. Lastly, provide one strategy to limit the amount of times you sit for one consecutive hour.

Times in one day spent sitting for at least one consecutive hour	In one week, how many minutes would be reduced from your life expectancy?
	(e.g., 4 times per day × 7 days per week = 28 times per week. 28 times per week × 22 minutes per time = 616 minutes)
Provide one strategy for decreasing the amount of times you sit for one consecutive hour.	

The Evolution of the Sedentary Lifestyle

Life is very different today than 100 years ago! Transportation, work, entertainment, and recreation have changed dramatically. There is much more technology available! The Internet, cars, airplanes, food preservation, food preparation, and seemingly endless amounts resources are all more available to people. Today, physical activity, in many ways, has been outsourced from daily life. This is certainly a major health concern in the United States as physical inactivity accounts for nearly 1 out of every 10 deaths.[2] In other words, up to 10 percent of deaths today can be linked to physical inactivity! Is it likely that one out of every 10 deaths was linked to physical inactivity generations ago? Probably not!

Turning back the clock, not that long ago, people had to be physically active to thrive and survive in society. People lived in a predominantly agrarian society. This meant people had to wake up in the morning and tend to crops, animals, and work to prepare each meal they consumed. This is very different from the lifestyle today! Many people cannot imagine waking up at the crack of dawn and working for two hours just to be able to prepare breakfast and get everything in-line to prepare the other meals in the day as well. Beyond preparing for meals, people had to constantly work to maintain food stores for the non-growing seasons, gather wood to heat the home in the winter, and constantly maintain equipment. Life generations ago required an immense amount of physical work nearly every day! Also the temperature in the home was dissimilar. Today, people have the luxury of living in environments with heat and air conditioning both of which maintain a fairly constant temperature in their environment. This was not the case generations ago. People were forced to burn more calories in order to maintain their body temperatures at 98.6 degrees. Today, not so much! Plain and simple, the lifestyle people lived generations ago resulted in the expenditure of far more calories than the average person expends today.

Staying in the days of yesteryear, people worked much harder to get from point A to point B. How did people get from their house to the local market? Even further back, how did the pioneers migrate deep into the American frontier? The answer to these questions, in many cases, was by walking. Sure, people may have occasionally had the luxury of riding by horse, wagon, carriage, or train, but ultimately the primary mode of transportation was walking. How about today? How do people get around? People today travel by car, by bus, and by airplane. It is fairly rare that people in today's society are forced into transportation by foot; it's definitely not the norm. In days past, travel by foot was indeed the norm. Just by walking as the primary mode of transportation, people generations ago expended more calories and were more physically active in everyday life.

How about entertainment and recreation? Today, people have numerous options for entertainment and recreation. Going to a movie, a baseball game, or concert are all forms of entertainment in today's society. Aside from these activities being fun and enjoyable, what do these activities all have in common? The answer is they are sedentary forms of entertainment. Another form of entertainment among the younger population is playing video games. Once again, this is a sedentary behavior. Even some of the leisure activities people do in today's society are not activities that would be considered moderate intensity. Playing a round of golf is great, but it often involves riding in a cart. When it comes to entertainment and recreation, there exists a tremendous opportunity to incorporate forms of physical activity. Simply put, people need to make the conscious decision to find forms of entertainment and recreation which require more movement and less sedentary time.

In many cases, there is no avoiding sedentary behavior. In today's society, more and more people make a living by pounding away at the keyboard behind a desk. Thinking of the average workday, a person wakes up, sits in a car for 30 or more minutes during the morning commute, sits for 8 hours behind a desk, sits in a car for 30 or more minutes on the drive home, and then lounges back in the recliner for 3 hours before going to bed. Rise and repeat! This is a very destructive lifestyle, even if someone adheres to a well-designed exercise program.

To make this more relatable, what many college students aspire to do in their professional careers has an impact on long-term health. Many of the jobs college students aspire to pursue upon graduation include jobs in what are known as STEM fields. STEM stands for science, technology, engineering, and mathematics. Jobs that require knowledge or skills in one or more of these areas typically are higher paying jobs. So one can see why students pursue such careers. However, from a health standpoint, jobs in science, technology, engineering, and mathematics can impose long-term health risks. The reason is that these jobs often involve prolonged periods of sitting and sedentary behavior. Even non-STEM jobs like those in law and business involve prolonged periods of sitting and sedentary behavior. Therefore, college students need to develop strategies for avoiding prolonged periods of sitting once they enter the workforce. These strategies most certainly do not require a career change. That is definitely not the message here at all! The message is college students need to develop habits of physical activity beyond just going to the gym three to five days per week. Failing to do so will wash out many of the health benefits gained from adhering to an exercise program.

VOICES FROM CAMPUS 5.1

Bryan

I am a mechanical engineering major and I just finished my sophomore year of college. This is a big moment in my college years because I am currently doing my first co-op for a large company in Indiana that specializes in designing, developing, and manufacturing turbines for jet engines. The co-op is awesome. I get to draft the blueprints for new turbine designs and I get to test them through computer modeling. The only downside to my co-op is that I sit for such long periods of time. I actually found myself getting winded from walking up my apartment stairs, and I think I am getting out of shape and becoming unhealthy. So during my lunch break a few days ago, I read some articles that suggested sitting can be worse for my health than smoking. I chose the career path of a mechanical engineer because I am good at math and I want to make great money. Now I am concerned that my career may actually kill me.

Given my concern, I spoke to a health coach at my co-op company. I told the coach my concerns and even asked if I should change career paths. The health coach laughed and said, "You shouldn't change career paths just because the job requires lots of time behind a computer! You should change how you approach your job instead." I had no clue what this meant, so I had to ask her to clarify. She then suggested that I get a standing desk and go for a walk to the bathroom or water cooler every 30 minutes. She explained this helps prevent the adverse health effects of sitting down. I am awfully glad I spoke to a health coach! If not for her I may have switched majors. I can't wait to get my standing desk and continue pushing through in a career I will love!

Evolution of Sedentary Behavior

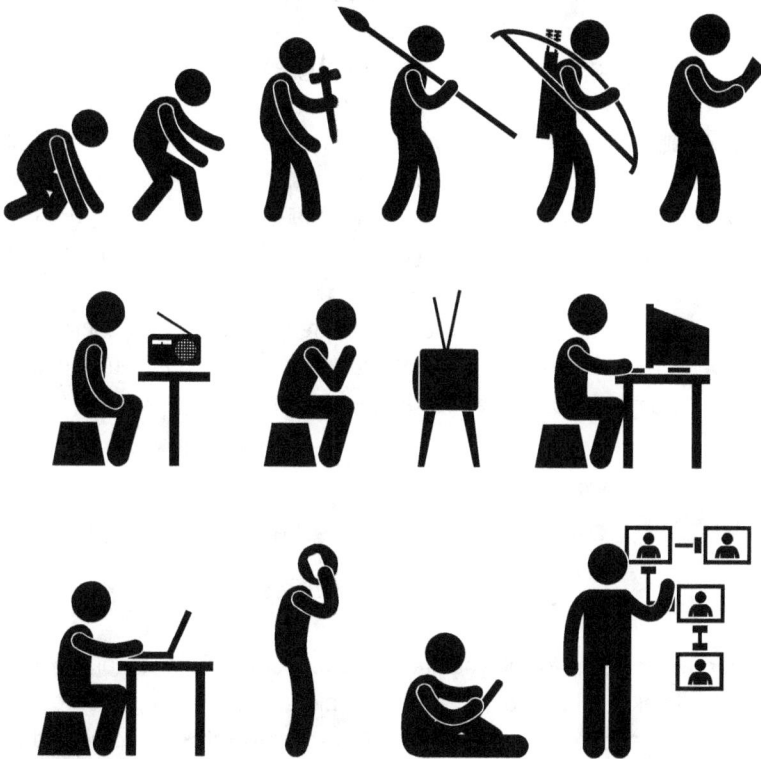

5.2: Getting More Physical Activity

To this point in Chapter 5, the overwhelming theme has been to complement regular exercise with other forms of physical activity. Now it is time to focus on choosing physical activities. Choosing physical activities to complement an exercise program is actually far easier than designing an exercise program from scratch. Which is easier: figuring out exercise frequency, intensity, time, and type or scheduling a round of golf in which everybody walks and carries their own golf bag? So the process for choosing physical activities is rather simplistic. Furthermore, the process of picking physical activities can prove to be rather enjoyable. The opportunities for getting in extra physical activity are literally endless! Physical activities can come in many forms and, in many cases, can be easily built into everyday routines. The one caveat in incorporating physical activities is overcoming many common barriers, like a perceived lack of time. Overcoming barriers to physical activity will be discussed in the next section.

In review, physical activity is defined as any bodily movement which elevates metabolic demands such as heart rate, breathing, and caloric expenditure. With this in mind, many pursuits would be considered a form of physical activity. Playing racquetball, backyard football, or working in the garden are all forms of physical activity. For instance, the simple and everyday task of walking is a great option. Walking would be considered physical activity. Walking is most definitely a bodily movement, and even a leisurely stroll can elicit caloric expenditures two to three times greater than just sitting down and watching television. Just incorporating 30 minutes of brisk walking per day has a tremendously positive influence on overall health. In general, finding time to incorporate 30 minutes of any moderate physical activity has tremendous benefits.

YOUR TURN 5.3

Physical Activities

Directions: At this point, you are well aware of the definition of physical activity. Thinking about your everyday life, please list five things you do that would be considered a physical activity. Next, list five physical activities that you are currently not doing that you could include in your everyday life. Lastly, explain why each of these activities would be considered a physical activity.

Physical activities you currently do	Why are these considered physical activities?	Physical activities you are not doing, but could do	Why are these considered physical activities?
1.			
2.			
3.			
4.			
5.			

Incorporating More Physical Activity Into Everyday Life

It is no secret that increasingly more and more jobs today require long hours of what would be considered sedentary behaviors. This point has certainly been explained in this chapter. However, this book has not yet suggested how people might attack this problem. From reading this chapter, one may assume that quitting a job or even changing careers might be an option. The problem is these are not very good options. Quitting a job or changing careers just for the sake of getting more physical activity is a lot like buying a shoe store to get free shoes. It makes little to no sense. Therefore, it is far more important to develop reasonable strategies for incorporating physical activity into daily routines.

Thinking about an average workday, a person may arrive to work at 9 a.m. and immediately sit behind a computer, check emails, and then begin to run financial analyses for the company for the next several hours. A reasonable solution to this sedentary "problem" would be to break up that period of sedentary behavior with just one minute of physical activity. Frequent breaks in sedentary time, of just one to four minutes per break, are associated with far better health outcomes than if sedentary times persist. These breaks in sedentary time do not have to involve overly intense physical activity. In fact, just standing up and taking a walk over to the water cooler or to the restroom would be considered a break in sedentary time. These types of breaks, though very short and light in intensity, are actually very beneficial to overall health. A recent study found that those who frequently broke up periods of sedentary time had an average waist circumference of 5.9 cm less than those who did not break up sedentary time.[3] Such a small effort incorporated into an average workday can definitely have lasting positive benefits. After reviewing the research, it appears there are few concrete recommendations for how often sedentary times should be broken up, but in general, people should try to break up sedentary times every 20 to 30 minutes.

Another method to consider is altering a work desk. Everyone is well aware of what a typical desk looks like, but there are new desks that can replace the old. Standing and treadmill desks are fairly recent innovations and are used frequently by people in the workplace. These desks have many designs—some can be rather inexpensive, while others are more on the pricey end. Using a standing desk at work or while studying has many reported benefits, and it is generally accepted that using a standing desk instead of a sitting desk has a positive influence on overall health. However, the treadmill desk may provide a bit more benefit as using a treadmill desk requires more effort and thus more calories will be expended. Also people could consider sitting on a stability ball as opposed to a desk chair. Sitting on a stability ball causes the muscles of the abdomen to constantly contract to hold the spine in an upright position. These contractions have been shown to reduce low back pain and improve core strength. Moreover, more calories are burned when sitting on a stability ball than when sitting in a common desk chair.

Now that techniques for incorporating physical activity into the time spent at work have been discussed, attention can be paid to other daily changes that can increase physical activity. One of the simplest forms of physical activity is walking. Walking is often an underrated form of physical activity, but it can be very effective at improving health and it's super easy to do more of in everyday life. Almost everybody has been in a car when the driver has driven up and down the lanes of a parking lot looking for the closest parking spot. This is actually a very lazy habit and people are missing a golden opportunity to get more physical activity. Instead of parking in the front of the lot, and wasting time looking for that closer spot, parking in the back of the lot and walking into the building is healthier. Here, people may get up to an extra 1/8 of a mile or more of walking per visit to work, the grocery store, or a shopping mall. Assuming people go to work five times a week, to the grocery store once a week, and to the shopping mall once a week, this provides no less than seven opportunities to increase the amount of physical activity. If each time this adds 100 yards worth of walking from the car and 100 yards walking back to the car, then that adds up to nearly 1 mile extra of walking per week. This additional walking would burn around 100 extra calories per week. When adding this up over the course of a year, it equates to nearly two pounds of weight loss. Though people may not notice such a small change in weight, this extra physical activity can help prevent obesity and many other adverse health effects.

Another lazy habit is not taking the stairs when possible. Escalators and elevators certainly make life easier, but easier is not always better. Taking the stairs whenever possible will definitely help improve health. Going back to the parking lot example, not every destination has a parking lot, some have parking garages. Instead of parking on the bottom floor, go all the way to the top and take the stairs into the building and back to the car. Once again this is a simple way to get more physical activity and it is far more beneficial to overall health than parking on the bottom floor and taking the elevator. In total, combining the example of always parking in the back of the parking lot, always taking the stairs, and always parking on the top floor of a parking garage represents a significant increase in physical activity levels over the course of a week, a year, and a lifetime. And the benefits to health are substantial!

"Standing Desk"

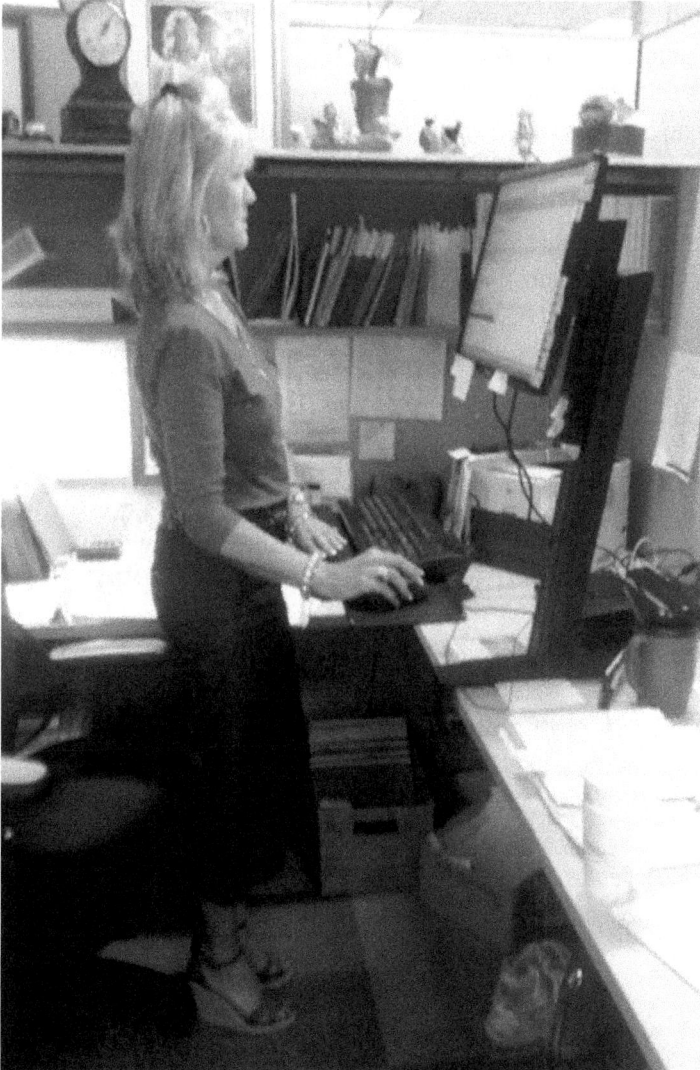

Beyond the simplistic methods of increasing physical activity in the routine day, there are many other options for increasing overall physical activity. Options do not just have to be playing pickup games of basketball and other sports. There are many more options and methods out there. One very useful method could be to introduce new hobbies. Hobbies like golf, gardening, hiking, and hunting all can be forms of physical activity. A typical golf course is about 5,000 yards in length. Golfers with accurate shots are likely to walk about three miles each time they golf. Golfers with less accurate shots walk even farther! Gardening also has the potential to be very physical and is often a recommended form of physical activity for elderly citizens. Much movement is required in gardening. There is watering, digging, filling, pruning, and spraying. Hiking is a very obvious form of physical activity as it consists of walking, but it can be particularly challenging if there are changes in terrain and hills. Hunting may not seem like a form of physical activity, but walking into proper position in the open fields, swamps, and woodlands can be very taxing. Also if hunting is done with a group, people may take turns walking the area trying to stir up game. Finding forms of physical activity is an opportunity to get creative!

YOUR TURN 5.4

Identifying and Changing Lazy Habits

Directions: There are many habits that we have that may be considered lazy. These lazy habits may actually be habits that get rid of the opportunity for increasing physical activity such as parking in the closest parking spot and always using the elevator. Please identify five lazy habits you currently have. Then explain how you could change each of these habits into behaviors that increase your physical activity. Try not to use the examples of the parking lot and stairs. Think critically and be creative. Lastly, do you feel your current lazy habits are detrimental to YOUR health? Why or why not?

Lazy Habits	How could you turn this lazy habit into an opportunity for increasing physical activity?
1.	
2.	
3.	
4.	
5.	

Are your current lazy habits detrimental to YOUR health? Why or why not?

Strategies for Overcoming Barriers to Getting More Physical Activity

Virtually anybody can come up with reasons for not getting more physical activity on a daily basis. Many of these reasons are legitimate. Barriers like one's social surroundings, motivation, and limited time and resources are legitimate and may result in not getting the needed amounts of physical activity for improving health. However, these barriers do not have to be the reason that physical activity is not completed. There are many strategies for overcoming these barriers.

One's social surroundings can be a barrier. Some students may have friends and family who do not value physical activity and do not desire to take it up. In college, there are endless opportunities for meeting new people. Mingling with new people in class, taking new classes to meet new people, or joining a fitness group and finding new role models are all possible. These strategies can be very beneficial toward overcoming social barriers that may prevent someone from getting much needed physical activity. Also college is a time when inevitably young men and women will go on dates. It would be fun and beneficial to go on dates that require physical activity. Going bowling, dancing, rowing, rock climbing, or hiking are all fun and healthy dating ideas.

At some point, almost all college students face a period of time when they lose motivation. For whatever reason, this appears to be commonplace. It is helpful to stick to a schedule and routine. So building in times for physical activity is very helpful. For instance, students could carve out time in between classes to go for a stroll across campus or walk the stairs of the football stadium. Another great strategy for overcoming a lack of motivation is by having a partner or friend who can serve as someone to do physical activity with or simply add accountability. Additionally, people can often try to remind themselves of all of the benefits they will gain by pushing through and doing more physical activity.

A lack of resources is definitely a legitimate barrier to getting physical activity. A lack of money and access to safe areas can hinder opportunities to get physical activity. However, they are not complete barriers and can be overcome. Choosing physical activities that require little or no money is a good financial strategy. Activities like walking and taking the stairs are free forms of physical activity. If safety is a concern, it is very useful to perform physical activities in well-lit areas, during daylight hours, and with a group of friends.

YOUR TURN 5.5

Overcoming Barriers

Directions: There are many barriers that may prevent us from getting enough physical activity. Please identify five barriers you may be currently facing that could limit your physical activity. Then provide a simple strategy for overcoming each barrier. Lastly, which barrier do you feel is the most difficult to overcome and explain why you feel this is so.

Barriers	How could you overcome this barrier?
1.	
2.	
3.	

4.	
5.	

Which barrier is the most difficult for you to overcome? Explain why.

5.3: The Take Away

- In order to maximize the effectiveness of an exercise program and maintain all health benefits gained through regular exercise, additional physical activity is required.

- Sedentary behaviors are behaviors that burn less than 1.5 times the calories required to stay alive.

- Prolonged engagement in sedentary behaviors can lead to developing metabolic syndrome and increased risk of cardiovascular disease and type 2 diabetes.

- Prolonged sedentary behavior such as watching television, playing video games, or sitting can wash away the benefits achieved through regular exercise.

- Sitting for long periods of time can be more detrimental to overall health than smoking.

- Young adults should focus on developing strategies for limiting sedentary behaviors and prolonged sitting.

- Breaking up sedentary time at work by doing light, one-to-four-minute bouts of physical activity can limit the adverse health effects of prolonged sedentary behaviors.

- Using innovative strategies like a standing desk, a walking treadmill desk, and sitting on a stability ball at work or while studying can have lasting positive health benefits and outcomes.

- Incorporating simple physical activities into everyday life like parking in the back of a parking lot and always using the stairs helps ward off adverse health consequences like gaining weight.

- Choosing physical activities is an opportunity to be creative. An excellent strategy for getting more physical activity is by developing new hobbies like golfing, gardening, hiking, or hunting.

- There are many barriers to getting physical activity. These barriers can be overcome through several strategies including teaming up with a partner, joining new social groups, going on dates that are more physically demanding, and limiting physical activities which require increased monetary expenses.

References

1. Biswas, A., Oh, P. I., Faulkner, G. E., Bajaj, R. R., Silver, M. A., Mitchell, M. S., & Alter, D. A. (2015). Sedentary time and its association with risk for disease incidence, mortality, and hospitalization in adults: A systematic review and meta-analysis. *Annals of Internal Medicine, 162*(2), 123–132.
2. Danaei, G., Ding, E. L., Mozaffarian, D., Taylor, B., Rehm, J., Murray, C. J., & Ezzati, M. (2011). The preventable causes of death in the United States: Comparative risk assessment of dietary, lifestyle, and metabolic risk factors. *PLoS Medicine, 6*(4). doi:10.1371/annotation/0ef47acd-9dcc-4296-a897-872d182cde57
3. Healy, G. N., Dunstan, D. W., Salmon, J., Cerin, E., Shaw, J. E., Zimmet, P. Z., & Owen, N. (2008). Breaks in sedentary time. *Diabetes Care, 31*(4), 661–666.
4. Healy, G. N., Matthews, C. E., Dunstan, D. W., Winkler, E. A., & Owen, N. (2011). Sedentary time and cardio-metabolic biomarkers in US adults: NHANES 2003–06. *European Heart Journal, 32*(5), 590–597.
5. Katzmarzyk, P. T., Church, T. S., Craig, C. L., & Bouchard, C. (2009). Sitting time and mortality from all causes, cardiovascular disease, and cancer. *Medicine and Science in Sports Exercise, 41*(5), 998–1005.
6. Pate, R. R., O'Neill, J. R., & Lobelo F. (2008). The evolving definition of "sedentary." *Exercise and Sports Sciences Review, 36*(4), 173–178.
7. Thorp, A. A., Healy, G. N., Owen, N., Salmon, J., Ball, K., Shaw, J. E., Zimmet, P. Z., & Dunstan, D. W. (2010). Deleterious associations of sitting time and television viewing time with cardiometabolic risk biomarkers. *Diabetes Care, 33*(2), 327–334.
8. Van der Ploeg, H. P., Chey, T., Korda, R. J., Banks, E., & Bauman, A. (2012). Sitting time and all-cause mortality risk in 222 497 Australian adults. *Archives of Internal Medicine, 172*(6), 494–500.
9. Veerman, J. L., Healy, G. N., Cobiac, L. J., Vos, T., Winkler, E. A. H., Owen, N., & Dunstan, D. W. (2012). Television viewing time and reduced life expectancy: A life

table analysis. *British Journal of Sports Medicine, 46*(13), 927–930. doi:10.1136/bjsm.2011.085662

10. Wilmot, E. G., Edwardson, C. L., Achana, F. A., Davies, M. J., Gorely, T., Gray, L. J., Khunti, K., Yates, T., & Biddle, S. J. (2012). Sedentary time in adults and the association with diabetes, cardiovascular disease and death: Systematic review and meta-analysis. *Diabetologia, 55*(11), 2895–2905.

Image Credits

ALTERNATIVE EXERCISE PROGRAMS

I did not realize there are so many rules for exercising to stay healthy. Can't I do some exercising for fun?

U p until this point, this book has focused on many topics. Discussions ranging from the public health crisis as it relates to physical inactivity to the components of an exercise program have been presented. Even more, this text dove into basic human physiology, health, and the need for regular exercise. Terms like aerobic, resistance, flexibility, and neuromotor exercise have been mentioned and hashed out several times and examples of these types of exercises have been provided. While these concepts and terms are truly important and discussions of such are really needed to portray the overall message of this book, which is "exercise for improving health," readers may still have questions regarding exercise.

Readers may be questioning if there are other exercises and exercise programs available to them. From this text, readers may conclude that the only effective exercise programs available to them are those that involve typical fitness center cardio and weight equipment. What about the exercise programs and equipment being sold on television advertisements? What about all of the exercise classes available at the local recreation center? What about fitness video games? The reality is there are many forms of exercise that people can do to improve health. People do not have to be limited by the available equipment at the local gym, nor do they have to be limited by a complete dislike for traditional forms of exercise like running on a treadmill or lifting weights.

Given the countless alternative exercise programs that are available in today's society, the final chapter of this book will discuss a variety of those programs. Specifically, Chapter 6 will provide an overview of some of these programs. In doing so, the safety and effectiveness of those programs will be discussed. Finally, Chapter 6 will wrap up by giving final recommendations for those who are truly interested in exercising to improve health.

6.1: Alternative Exercise Programs

Alternative exercise programs can be defined in numerous ways. However, pinpointing a precise definition can be somewhat tricky. Exercise programs that many exercise professionals would consider "alternative" would be described by other exercise professionals as falling in line with the fundamentals of exercise program design. So for the purpose of this text, alternative exercise programs can be defined as any exercise program that does not conform to the general exercise recommendations for improving health. As a refresher these recommendations are a minimum of 30 minutes moderate aerobic exercise per day,

Boot Camp is an Alternative Exercise Program.

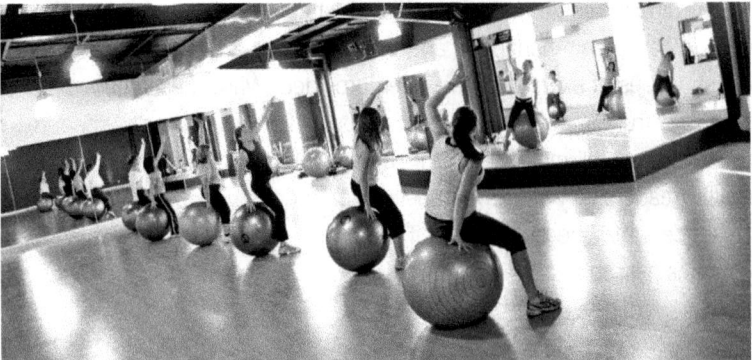

three days per week, plus two additional days of resistance exercise, performing one resistance exercise for each major muscle group. Also, physical activities that have been discussed in this book would not be considered an alternative exercise program. Remember, exercise is planned and structured with the goal of improving fitness while physical activities are not. So activities like walking, golfing, playing basketball, or gardening would not be considered alternative exercise programs.

OUR TURN 6.1

Alternative Exercise Programs

Directions: Now that you know the definition of an alternative exercise program, please list five alternative exercise programs that you have heard of. Then list two alternative exercise programs that you have done before. Lastly, list two alternative exercise programs that you think you would find enjoyable.

List five alternative exercise programs
1.
2.
3.
4.
5.

List two alternative exercise programs you have done before
1.
2.

List two alternative exercise programs you may find enjoyable
1.
2.

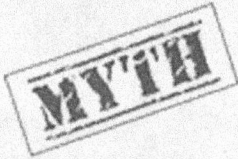

The American College of Sports Medicine publishes several exercise guidelines. Among these guidelines is the recommended exercise dose for improving health for healthy adults. These guidelines stem from years of research and are designed to help the most people posssible to improve their health and reduce the risk for developing many chronic diseases. However, these guidelines do not have to be the only exercise presciption. While research does show that these guidelines improve health, there are other exercise prescriptions that can improve health. As long as an exercise program is specific to individual goals and adequately stresses the physiological systems required for accomplishing goals, then that program will be effective. This means programs like Zumba, spinning, and CrossFit can help people improve their health. So if you do not like what the exercise recommendations for improving health have to offer, then you should choose another program that is specific, effective, and safe for meeting your goals.

The general exercise recommendations for improving health have been determined, through years of research, to be the most effective exercise method for eliciting the physiological adaptations needed for warding off disease. This, however, does not mean that adhering to these recommendations is the "be-all and end-all" way to evoke positive physiological adaptations. In some cases, depending on the person, alternative exercise programs may actually lead to more benefits than adhering to the exercise recommendations for improving health.

In 2017, researchers, healthcare professionals, and fitness experts are all aware that any form of exercise will likely lead to some positive benefit. The extent of the health benefits gained from completing alternative exercise programs is currently being debated. Also, given the limited research on many alternative exercise programs, additional concerns exist for the safety of such programs. Therefore, whenever people embark on an alternative exercise program they must be aware of the effectiveness and safety of the program.

Alternative exercise programs come in many forms and fashions. There are many fads, gimmicks, and false claims surrounding many alternative exercise programs. In addition to considering the safety and effectiveness of an alternative exercise program, the decision to choose an alternative exercise program in lieu of the exercise recommendations for improving health needs to be made with individual goals in mind. Alternative exercise programs, like traditional exercise programs, need to incorporate the basic principles of exercise program design. Therefore, the program must include movements and intensities that are specific for eliciting the adaptations needed to accomplish goals and have a strategy of progressive overload. The following sections are dedicated to discussing various alternative exercise programs.

CrossFit

CrossFit is a relatively new strength and conditioning program and is becoming an increasingly popular alternative exercise program. CrossFit emphasizes short, yet sustained, high-intensity bouts of exercise with little to no rest periods. Workouts in CrossFit contain both aerobic and resistance exercise qualities. Additionally, the exercises used in CrossFit are typically whole body and multi-joint exercises. CrossFit training is most commonly completed in classes or groups in what are called CrossFit gyms. CrossFit gyms are not your typical fitness facility. They are usually open indoor spaces and have nontraditional exercise equipment like battle ropes, tractor tires, sledgehammers, gymnastic rings, and free weights. Legitimate CrossFit classes are led by an exercise professional who is specially certified to instruct people in CrossFit training. A prerequisite for joining a CrossFit class must be that the instructor is certified. There are many instances of people claiming to be CrossFit instructors who are not properly trained nor certified. Ensuring that the instructor is certified in CrossFit is one of the best ways to avoid injury during CrossFit training.

REFERENCES:

Pescatello, L., Arena, R., Riebe, D., Thompson, P. D. (2013). ACSM's guidelines for exercise testing and prescription (4th ed.). Baltimore: Lippincott, Williams & Wilkins.

The hallmark of CrossFit is the "workout of the day." "Workouts of the day" consist of functional lifts such as the squat, deadlift, hang clean, snatch clean, and push press. These exercises could be classified as functional because they have a transferrable effect to improving a person's ability to carry out activities of daily living. As exercisers advance in CrossFit training and adapt to these functional exercises, more difficult exercises are added to the "workouts of the day." These advanced exercises can include pull-ups, tire flips, battle ropes, hitting tractor tires with sledgehammers, and gymnastic exercises using rings. Oftentimes the "workout of the day" is completed with an emphasis on finishing within the shortest amount of time possible. An example of this type of "workout of the day" is performing three sets of three different exercises. Here, the exercises may be the deadlift, push press, and pull-ups. Other "workouts of the day" may involve completing as many sets of a series of exercises as possible in 10 to 20 minutes.

There have been some studies that examined the benefits of CrossFit training. However, CrossFit training is very random in the exercises that are performed and from a research standpoint it is incredibly challenging to accurately compare CrossFit training to more traditional training programs. Despite this challenge, research has shown that CrossFit can be very beneficial to overall health. Adhering to a CrossFit program is associated with improvements in cardiorespiratory endurance, muscular strength, and body composition. Furthermore, improvements in some of the components of skill-related physical fitness have been observed in response to CrossFit training.

Given that CrossFit emphasizes high-intensity exercises that require a certain degree of skill, one of the biggest concerns many health and fitness professionals have with CrossFit is safety. A recent survey study showed that 73.5 percent of those participating in CrossFit sustained an injury during training.[1] Another recent survey study revealed an injury rate of 20 percent.[2] Though these two studies show a wide discrepancy in the injury rate for CrossFit participants, the reality is that the very nature of CrossFit has high potential to lead to injury. Injury to the knees, shoulders, and low back are fairly common in CrossFit. There are several considerations people can make to decrease the risk of injury during CrossFit training. The first has already been mentioned and that is to ensure the instructor is certified in CrossFit. A certified trainer in CrossFit is equipped with knowledge and skills needed to guide people in choosing the proper weight to be lifted and in instructing safe and proper techniques. The second is individuals must always use the

CrossFit Workout of the Day

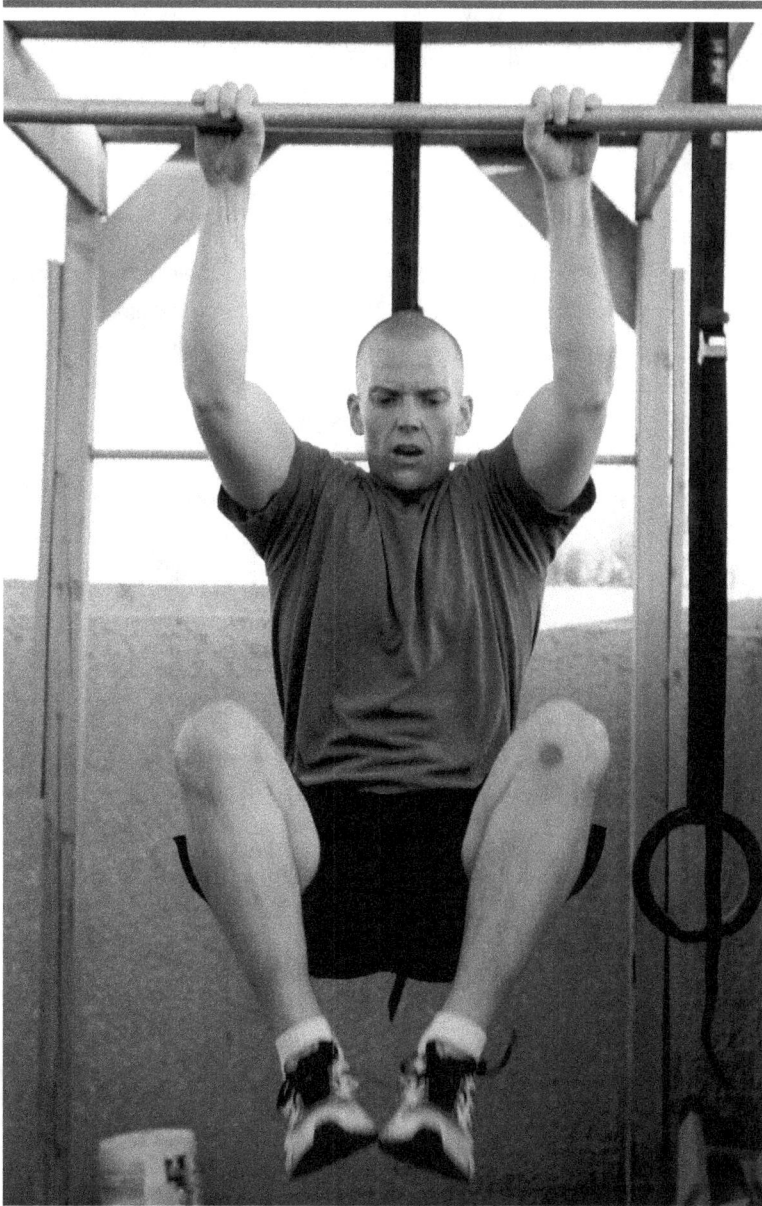

proper exercise techniques. Not executing CrossFit exercises with the proper mechanics will almost always lead to injury. Third, exercises should always start with low weights. Once the exercise is mastered, then weight can be added. Fourth, always have a spotter. A fifth concern is people should avoid exercising through pain and injury since this only makes injuries worse. Lastly, if a person has a history of injury or was previously inactive before starting CrossFit, it is wise to get medical clearance before beginning CrossFit training.

Overall CrossFit does appear to be an effective alternative exercise program. Improvements in all the components of health-related physical fitness can be achieved through CrossFit. However, it is a good idea to establish a baseline fitness level prior to beginning CrossFit. This does not mean people have to be in elite physical condition to do CrossFit; it means that it is not wise to go from the couch directly to CrossFit training. Starting with a moderately intense aerobic exercise program and resistance program will help people build up their fitness and exercise tolerance to the point that CrossFit can be a sustainable and viable alternative exercise program for improving health.

Plyometric Training

Plyometric exercise training is predominately used by athletes of various sports, though other populations may incorporate plyometric exercises into an exercise program. Plyometric training consists of exercises in which movements are quick and explosive. The idea behind these movements is to exert maximal force in the shortest amount of time. In physics, a force divided by time equals power. Therefore plyometric exercise training is essentially power training. In today's world of sports, most athletes need to be both strong and quick. Consider offensive lineman in the NFL—they must be strong to move an opponent off of the line of scrimmage, but in order for the offensive lineman's strength to be effective it needs to be exerted quickly. Otherwise a defensive lineman or linebacker will absorb the initial force and simply slide off of the offensive lineman and tackle the running back. Also, a basketball player needs to be able to grab a rebound. It does basketball players little good to jump high if they cannot jump quickly, or else, the opponent will grab the rebound first. There are countless other examples of athletes needing power for elite performance. The tennis serve, the golf tee shot, the shot put, the baseball swing, the softball pitch, the soccer kick, and the list goes on and on. For these reasons, it is easy to see why athletes use plyometric exercises as a part of a strength and conditioning program.

Plyometric exercises can be beneficial for other populations as well. For starters, plyometric exercises are very demanding. This means that plyometric exercises are good for increasing the amount of calories skeletal muscles burn at rest. So plyometric exercise training can be used to help maintain adequate body composition. But there are other benefits the general population can gain from plyometric exercise training as well. The very nature of plyometric exercises requires a certain degree of technical know-how and skill. The brain and nervous system must work in "overdrive" to send electrical signals back and forth in order to communicate where the body's limbs are in space. This means that plyometric exercises enhance what is known as proprioception. Proprioception can be defined as knowing where the body's limbs, joints, and muscles are in space. Balancing oneself requires signals sent to the brain and spinal cord from sensory nerves in the muscles and joints, photoreceptors in the eye, and sensory receptors in the inner ear. Take away one of those signals, for instance by closing the eyes, and balancing becomes exponentially more difficult. Therefore, a transferrable effect of plyometric training to everyday life would be that a person is less likely to suffer common injuries as a result of poor balance. All in all, plyometric exercise training can be good for improving overall health, if used correctly!

Balance Positions

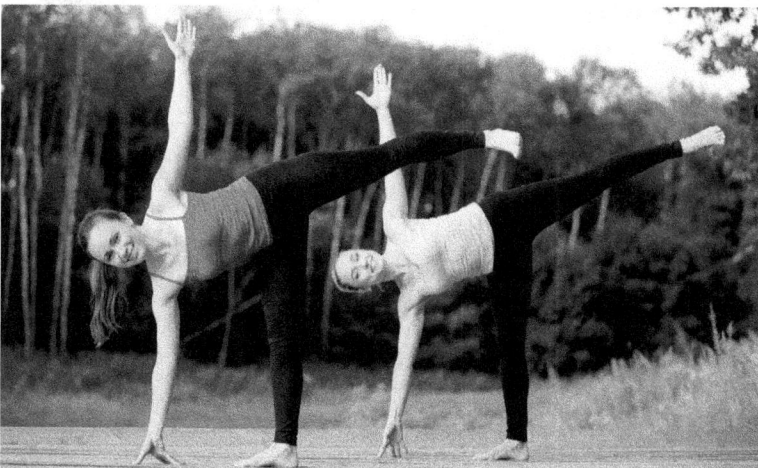

VOICES FROM CAMPUS 6.1

Nathan

I am a construction management major and I'm finishing up my junior year of college. This for me means on-the-job training! This really won't be my first time stepping foot onto a construction site though. I have helped my uncle Jimmy at his small company for years, but now I am going to be interning with the biggest construction company in the state! I am not really nervous about doing the job well at my internship because I have previous experience. However, I am terrified about what my new bosses will think of me. Ever hear about Murphy's Law? Well this applies to me big time! I am really good at my work, but boy am I clumsy. I fall all the time and too often find myself in the emergency room. I would really hate to fall on my new job and make a bad impression. So I really need to find a way to improve my balance.

I spoke to an exercise science professor in passing the other day and I mentioned my problem. He asked if I ever exercise. I said, "Yes, I am an avid gym-goer!" I exercise five times a week doing weight lifting and cardio. I am in good shape I must say! Anyway, the professor suggested I try plyometric training with one of the strength coaches in the athletic department. I had no idea what plyometric training was all about, but being curious and somewhat desperate to improve my balance I visited a strength coach.

The strength coach put me through all kinds of jumping exercises in addition to some pretty tough medicine ball sit-up routines. I absolutely loved this training. I feel like I am in much better shape. I have actually lost some weight and now can see my abs; beach season is going to be awesome this year! But on a serious note, I went to work for my uncle this weekend and I moved around so much better and never once lost my balance! I am very confident that I won't fall during my new job. I am on my way, hopefully to my dream job!

There are several examples of plyometric exercises. Box jumps, hurdle jumps, medicine ball throws, medicine ball sit-ups, and clapping push-ups are all common plyometric exercises. A hallmark of any plyometric exercise is that there are two key phases of movement. The first phase is called the eccentric phase. Here, a stretch is applied to the muscles that will contract to produce the movement required. An example would be a box jump. Before leaping up onto the box, an exerciser must squat down into approximately a quarter squat position. Here, the glutes and quads are stretched out. Once the muscles are stretched there is then stored energy in the tendons of those muscles, like a stretched rubber band. Then, phase two, the concentric or contraction phase occurs. Here the stored energy in the tendons is released, and snap! A more explosive movement occurs like snapping a rubber band. Also, during the eccentric phase of a plyometric exercise, receptors within the muscle are stretched. The stretching of these receptors induces a more powerful muscular contraction due to what is called a stretch reflex. So a plyometric exercise causes more powerful contractions in two ways. The first way is by taking advantage of stored energy within stretched tendons. The second way is by inducing the stretch reflex. It is a double shot of power! However, in order for these powerful contractions to occur, the stretch cannot be too great (e.g., like a catcher's squat) and the concentric phase needs to happen very quickly after the stretch. Otherwise the stored energy in the tendons dissipates and the stretch receptors in the muscle become desensitized. All movements in plyometric exercises must be performed with quickness in mind.

Box Jumps

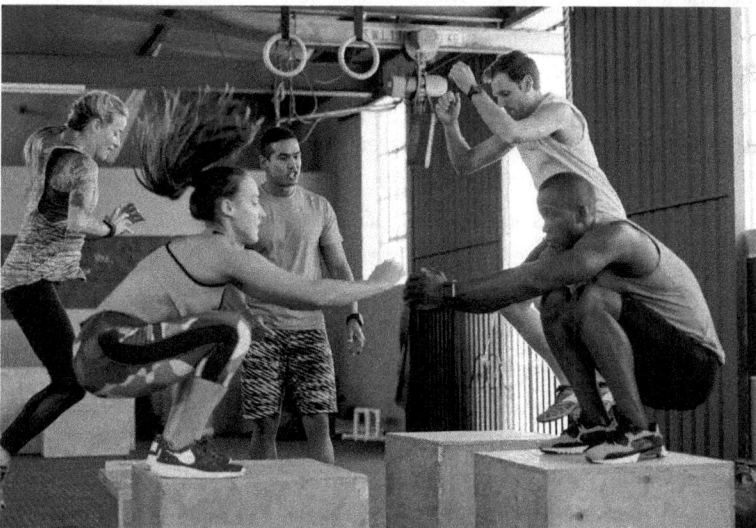

Plyometric exercise training does not come without risk. It is never recommended for beginning exercisers to take part in a plyometric exercise program as an alternative to a more traditional exercise program. There have been several recommendations as to when it is safe for someone to begin a plyometric program. Overall, the use of plyometric exercises should only be done if doing so is a necessity for achieving goals. Therefore, there needs to be a specific reason for doing plyometric exercise training. Other factors must be considered as well. Factors like age, fitness level, and past and current injury and medical histories must be taken into account. If a person has a history of musculoskeletal injuries, it is wise to seek medical clearance before beginning a plyometric program. Overall, there are two absolute requisites for plyometric training. First, plyometric training should only occur once someone has developed adequate strength and flexibility. Therefore, more traditional strength and flexibility programs need to be completed prior to ever attempting plyometric exercise training. Second, there must be supervision and an unyielding attention to correct technique. Like CrossFit, injuries are reduced when proper supervision and techniques are employed!

Yoga

Yoga is an ancient discipline designed to improve physical, mental, emotional, and spiritual dimensions of overall health. Yoga appears to have roots in religion and spirituality and many perform Yoga as a means of meditation. Beyond its religious roots, Yoga is often used in today's society as a form of exercise. As a form of exercise, Yoga requires exercisers to maintain "poses" for certain periods of time. These poses can range from those that require isometric muscular contractions aimed at improving muscular fitness to those that emphasize increasing range of motion. There are also varying intensities of Yoga exercises. Some Yoga poses are fairly simple and are intended for beginners while others are incredibly challenging. Furthermore, Yoga can be practiced in a variety of settings. Though most common in fitness centers, parks, and in the home, Yoga can be practiced in such settings as saunas (hot Yoga) in which the demands of poses are greatly increased.

There have been several studies showing excellent health benefits from participating in Yoga. One known, and arguably the most notable, benefit of Yoga is the reduction of stress. The reduction of stress stems from the chronic downregulation of the sympathetic nervous system. The sympathetic nervous system is the "fight or flight mechanism" of the human body. Increased activation of the sympathetic nervous system leads to increased heart rate, blood pressure, and even inflammation. By doing Yoga on a regular basis this downregulation of the sympathetic nervous system can be tied to decreases in the risk for cardiovascular disease, type 2 diabetes, and even certain cancers. Another notable benefit of Yoga is the reduction in musculoskeletal and joint pain. This reduction in pain is thought to occur as a result of increased muscular strength, particularly of the core, and improvements in overall flexibility. Yoga has also been used to help rehabilitate people from musculoskeletal injuries and even from the effects of cancer and cancer treatments. Recently, Yoga has been shown to help people overcome crippling drug and alcohol addictions.

There does need to be caution practiced when evaluating the health benefits of Yoga. Controlled and randomized studies are the most powerful studies for determining an intervention's effectiveness. With that said, it is rather difficult to perform such studies with Yoga. Therefore, the true effectiveness of Yoga will likely continue to be questioned. Even so, it does appear that Yoga is fairly effective at improving health. However, to ensure that the health benefits of Yoga are maximized, it is recommended that other

Yoga Poses

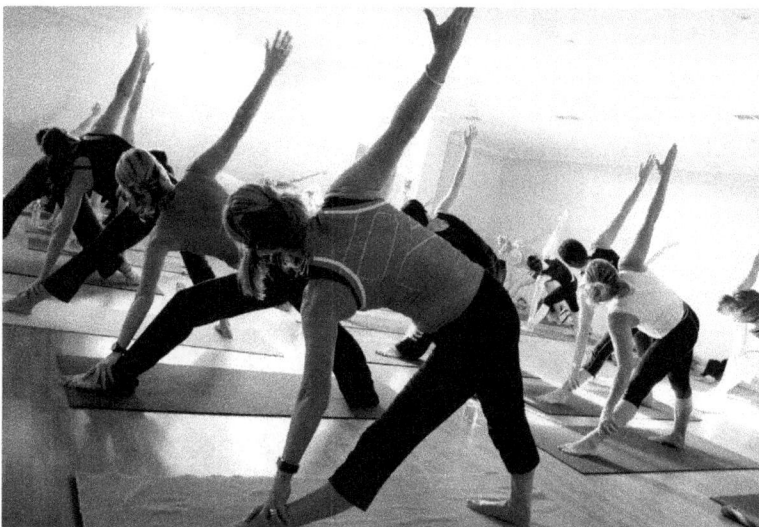

forms of exercise such as aerobic and resistance exercise be completed along with Yoga. Additionally, to ensure safety it is recommended that Yoga be completed under the supervision of a certified Yoga instructor and beginners should always master basic poses before moving on to advanced ones. Furthermore, Yoga performed in settings that increase the demands of the poses (e.g., hot Yoga) should only be performed by advanced exercisers and under supervision.

NFL Offensive Lineman

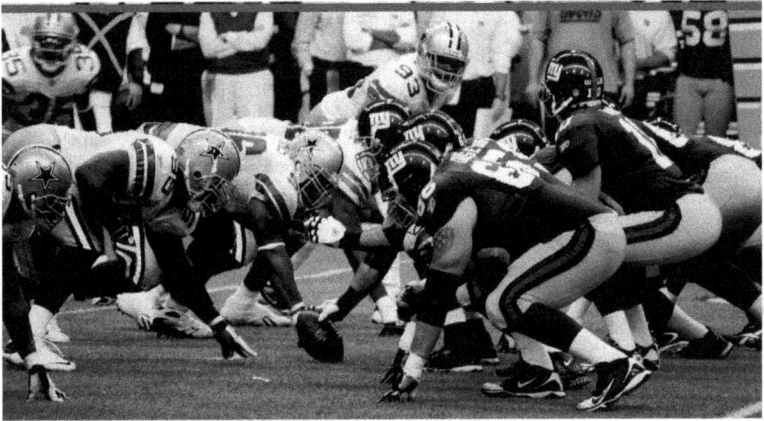

Group Exercise

Group exercise classes are increasing in their popularity. Classes like spinning, boot camp, aerobics, and Zumba are widely used by people to improve health. There are countless benefits to group exercise. First and foremost, participation in a well-designed group exercise class can help people dramatically improve the components of health-related physical fitness and improve overall health. Moreover, group exercise classes, to a large degree, hold people accountable for sustaining the positive behavior of incorporating exercise into weekly routines. Social cognitive theory is important here. The social cognitive theory claims that people can acquire knowledge, skills, attitudes, and beliefs from observing other people, who are similar to them, perform a certain behavior. An example of this is someone observing people in an exercise class and modeling that behavior. Overall, group exercise classes can help people increase their beliefs that they are capable of performing exercise on a regular basis. Furthermore, participating in a group exercise class is an excellent way to meet new people!

Group exercise classes can differ in terms of their overall effectiveness. For instance, a boot camp class may elicit benefits superior to a traditional aerobics class. The effectiveness of a group exercise class, in terms of eliciting positive health benefits, depends largely on the intensity of the exercise being performed. For instance, a spinning class may cause higher heart rates than a Zumba class. Therefore, like any alternative exercise program, people must choose a group exercise class that aligns with their goals. If a person's goal is improving muscular and cardiorespiratory endurance, then that person may choose boot camp or spinning.

Safety is always a priority when deciding to complete an alternative exercise program. Overall, the safety of group exercise programs is pretty good. Injuries are common when people perform exercises they are not capable of doing. So for beginners it is wise to choose a group exercise class that aligns with their skills and abilities. More advanced exercisers may choose group exercise classes like boot camp, which are significantly more intense. Similar to CrossFit, plyometric exercise training, and Yoga, group exercise classes should always be led and supervised by professionals who are certified in their exercise discipline.

Spinning is a Group Exercise Class

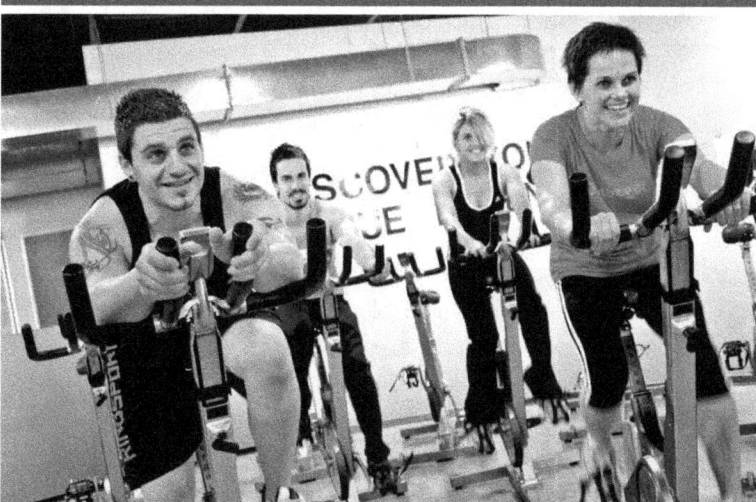

High-Intensity Interval Training

A major identified barrier for exercise participation in college students is a perceived lack of time. High-intensity interval training is an excellent method of exercise to combat this very barrier. High-intensity interval training is characterized by repeated bursts of relatively intense exercise separated by periods of rest or low-intensity exercise. In total, high-intensity interval training exercise sessions last between 10 and 30 minutes. High-intensity interval training can incorporate both aerobic and resistance exercises. Examples of high-intensity interval training are repeated sprints, weight lifting circuits, and some forms of CrossFit training.

There are countless health benefits that can be achieved through high-intensity interval training. Furthermore, in many cases these benefits are similar or even superior to those achieved through adherence to recommended exercise guidelines for improving health! This means optimal health benefits can be achieved with significantly less daily time requirement! These benefits include improvements in markers of cardiorespiratory endurance, body composition, blood glucose control, and fats in the blood. Also, adhering to a high-intensity interval training exercise program can greatly reduce a person's risk for developing cardiovascular disease, type 2 diabetes, and some cancers. What is more, high-intensity interval training has been shown to be a superior method for rehabilitating people with stable coronary artery disease and heart failure!

Oftentimes, high-intensity interval training programs involve performing load-bearing exercises at near maximal or maximal exercise intensities. These intensities may not be attainable for many populations and may increase the risk of injury. Therefore, high-intensity interval training should never be the beginning type of exercise program that people choose. There simply must be a baseline level of fitness that is established before doing a high-intensity interval training program. So, starting with a traditional exercise program will allow gradual increases in cardiorespiratory endurance and muscle fitness and thus make high-intensity interval training more tolerable. Also, it is absolutely essential that exercisers develop the proper exercise techniques before even considering high-intensity interval training. Failure to do so will almost certainly lead to injury. Lastly, important to ensuring safety, new exercisers should seek medical clearance from a medical doctor prior to beginning high-intensity interval training. The reason for this is simple: high-intensity exercise greatly increases the workload placed on the cardiovascular system and people should make certain they do not have an undiagnosed heart condition that can be exacerbated with high-intensity interval training.

Pilates

Although developed about 100 years ago Pilates has seen a recent increase in popularity since the 1980s. This form of exercise developed by Joseph Pilates was originally called "Contrology." The main principle is muscle control.

Pilates

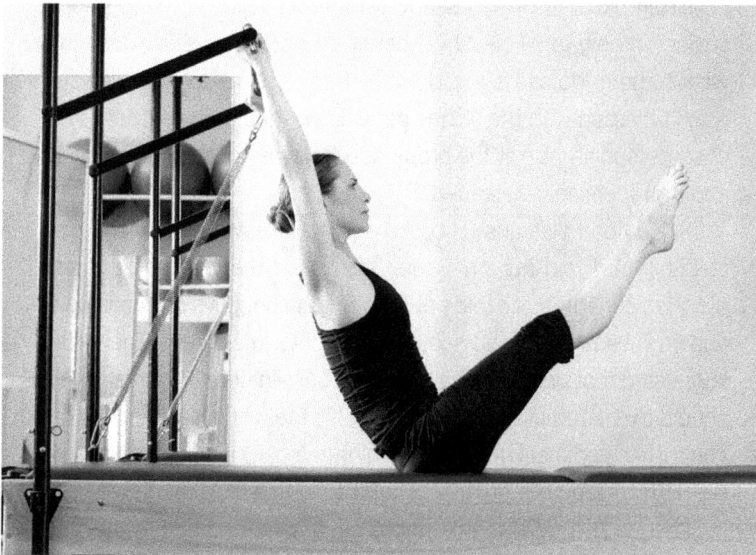

Pilates includes exercises generally done on a gym mat with a focus on core strength. The components of fitness developed by Pilates training include strength and flexibility. Other benefits include improved posture and mind/body awareness. Pilates does not develop cardiorespiratory fitness. Therefore, Pilates should be done in conjunction with at least three days of aerobic exercise per week.

One advantage of Pilates is adaptability. It has been used by elite athletes as well as beginners and individuals with various diseases. However, it is important that the instructor is qualified and knows all participants' limitations to make the class effective for all. The intensity of the class is in the middle range, but the muscles do get worked and potentially sore. Once the participants learn the workouts and proper techniques, the exercises can be done outside of formal classes and integrated into other training sessions.

VOICES FROM CAMPUS 6.2

Maggie

I am what many people would consider to be a gym rat and a nutrition freak. I love going to the gym and taking care of my body for a number of reasons. See, it is my goal to one day be a primary care physician. And, the way I see it, if I am going to be giving people advice on how to be healthy, I better be healthy myself. I don't just want to be a "do as I say and not as I do" type of doctor. Anyway, I wasn't blessed with the skinny gene. Even though I exercised like a crazy person and ate all the proper foods, I was not at my goal weight and had seemingly plateaued.

Since I had plateaued, I broke down and saw a personal trainer at the gym. I told her my issue. She asked me what my exercise program consisted of. I told her I run for one hour five days per week and on Tuesdays and Thursdays I lift weights, lots of reps! The trainer suggested that because I have a good baseline level of fitness that I should try HIIT training. I asked, "What is the world is HIIT training?" The trainer said that HIIT stood for high-intensity interval training and that HIIT training is a great way to take my fitness to the next level.

I began HIIT training with my trainer two months ago. It has been such an incredible challenge, and I love it! She has me doing intervals of all-out sprints on the cycle, treadmill, and rower. She even has me do weight lifting circuits on my lifting days. The pounds just seemed to melt right off of me. I went from 25 percent body fat down to 18 percent. I feel healthy, I look healthy, and I am healthy. The power of HIIT is nuts! I would suggest to any gym rat that is not doing HIIT to give it a shot, it sure helped me!

6.2: Final Recommendations for Choosing an Alternative Exercise Program

While adhering to the national exercise recommendations for improving health is shown to improve the components of health-related physical fitness and optimally decrease the risk for developing numerous and preventable chronic diseases, there are many alternative exercise programs that may offer similar benefits. It is of utmost importance that people evaluate two key aspects of any alternative exercise program: safety and effectiveness.

Exercise can do no good for anyone if it results in injury. Not only can injuries decrease a person's ability to exercise, injuries can limit the ability to carry out the functions of everyday living. Further, certain exercise programs may be so intense they cause complications from undiagnosed illnesses like cardiovascular disease. Therefore, before beginning an alternative exercise program, people should check to make sure instructors are certified, that they themselves are physically capable of performing the exercises, and that technique is always prioritized over results. As for safety, it is always a good idea to get a medical check-up prior to beginning an alternative exercise program.

The second aspect of an alternative exercise program that must be evaluated is effectiveness. There are so many gimmick exercise programs that are either ineffective or have not been studied. A prime example of this is the advertisement of certain exercise products. These products, in many cases, are not studied and the claimed benefits of these products may be far-fetched or even fabricated. For example, people cannot spot reduce fat; however, there are certain products that claim this can be done. So there is good reason to be cautious and approach exercise products and programs with a degree of skepticism. The best way to ensure that alternative exercise programs are effective is to research the program being considered. Google Scholar is an excellent search engine for looking up studies on alternative exercise programs. Also, when people look at studies they should always check in the "methods" section of the study to determine whether the study was a randomized control trial. Additionally, the very nature of an alternative exercise program must align with initial exercise goals. For instance, if a person seeks to improve muscular strength, then cycling class may not be a viable alternative exercise program. People must always assess the specificity of any exercise program for meeting individual goals.

YOUR TURN 6.2

Evaluating Alternative Exercise Programs

Directions: Now that you know you need to consider the specificity, safety, and effectiveness of an alternative exercise program before choosing to do it, please think of **one** alternative exercise program that may meet your fitness goals. First, what is your number one fitness goal? Now, use the search engine of your choice to research five health benefits of the exercise program. Then, list three ways to ensure your safety during that program. Lastly, explain whether you believe the alternative exercise program will help you meet your goal.

What is your alternative exercise program?
1.

What is your number one fitness goal?
1.

List five known health benefits of the program
1.
2.
3.
4.
5.

List three ways you can ensure your safety during this program
1.
2.
3.

> **Do you believe this alternative exercise program will help you meet your fitness goal? Why or why not?**

Lastly, people should choose exercise programs that they enjoy. This is a very critical decision. Exercise should not be perceived as miserable; it should be perceived as fun. Some people like running up stadium stairs while others are completely repulsed by the mere thought of running, and that is fine. There are exercises for everyone! If a person likes to dance, perhaps Zumba will be an effective alternative exercise program. If someone loves being in the water, maybe swimming and water aerobics is the ticket. The point is this: if people do not like an exercise program, then they will not continue to do it! Everyone should find an exercise program that is enjoyable and keep at, because any exercise program is better than no exercise program. Good luck and happy exercising!

6.3: The Take Away

- Any exercise program that does not conform to the general exercise recommendations for improving health can be considered an alternative exercise program.
- There are many alternative exercise programs that are available to people.
- When choosing an alternative exercise program people must evaluate the program for safety, effectiveness, and the specificity of achieving goals.
- Safety is improved when people have a baseline level of fitness, exercise under the supervision of a certified professional, always pay attention to exercise technique, and seek medical clearance before beginning an alternative exercise program.

- To evaluate the effectiveness of an alternative exercise program people should research the program. Research on alternative exercise programs can be found through search engines like Google Scholar.

- People should always choose exercises and exercise programs they enjoy. If people enjoy an exercise program, they are more likely to stick with it.

YOUR TURN 6.3

Personal Exercise Program Schedule

Using the SMART Goals, FITT-VP principle, and other concepts learned from this book as well as the **Your Turn** exercises, complete your personalized exercise program schedule on this form. Perhaps while reading this book you have tried some new exercises and found some you liked and disliked. Now is the time to take all the information you have learned and record it. This will be the program you will begin to follow, but remember that this program is fluid and adjustments should always be considered due to changes in goals, strengths and weaknesses, and likes and dislikes.

There are only seven days in a week, so consider how to use your time wisely. Prioritize your exercise choices and develop a weekly training schedule. As discussed you should have a minimum of three cardiorespiratory workouts, two resistance training workouts, and two flexibility workouts per week. You can do more than one in one day, especially for flexibility. And remember to save some time for rest and recovery (at least one or two days per week)!

Monday
Type of activity(ies) or exercise class _____

Tuesday
Type of activity(ies) or exercise class _____

Wednesday
Type of activity(ies) or exercise class _____

Thursday

Type of activity(ies) or exercise class _____

Friday

Type of activity(ies) or exercise class _____

Saturday

Type of activity(ies) or exercise class _____

Sunday

Type of activity(ies) or exercise class _____

References

1. Hak, P. T., Hodzovic, E., & Hickey, B. (2013). The nature and prevalence of injury during CrossFit training. *Journal of Strength and Conditioning Research.* doi:10.1519/JSC.0000000000000318
2. Weisenthal, B. M., Beck, C. A., Maloney, M. D., DeHaven, K. E., & Giordano, B. D. (2014). Injury rate and patterns among CrossFit athletes. *Orthopaedic Journal of Sports Medicine, 2*(4). doi:10.1177/2325967114531177

Image Credits

APPENDIX

WHERE TO TURN— ADDITIONAL RESOURCES

In Print

Brown L. E. (ed). (2017). *Strength Training*. Champaign, IL: Human Kinetics.

Broussal-Derval, A. & Ganneau, S. (2017). The Modern Art of High Intensity Training. Champaign, IL: Human Kinetics.

Bushman, B. A. (ed). (2017). *ACSM's Complete Guide to Fitness and Health*. Champaign, IL: Human Kinetics.

LaReine C. (2014). Weight Training For Dummies. New York, NY: John Wiley & Sons.

Hoeger, W. W. K., Hoeger, S. A., Hoeger, C. I. & Fawson, A.L. (2017). *Lifetime Physical Fitness and Wellness: A Personalized Program*. Boston, MA: Cengage Learning.

Matthews, J. (2016). *Stretching to Stay Young*. Berkeley, CA: Althea Press.

Naternicola, N. L. (2015). Fitness Steps to Success. Champaign, IL: Human Kinetics.

On the Web

American Heart Association. (2017). Physical Activity. http://www.heart.org/HEARTORG/HealthyLiving/PhysicalActivity/Physical-Activity_UCM_001080_SubHomePage.jsp

American Heart Association. (2015). Stretching and Flexibility Exercises. https://www.heart.org/HEARTORG/Conditions/More/CardiacRehab/Stretching-and-Flexibility-Exercises_UCM_307383_Article.jsp

Howard, N. (2011). 8 Exercises for Better Balance. http://www.sparkpeople.com/blog/blog.asp?post=8_exercises_for_better_balance

Office of Disease Prevention and Health Promotion. (2017). Physical Activity Guidelines. https://health.gov/paguidelines/

The Walking Site. (2017). The Walking Site. http://www.thewalkingsite.com/

Waehner, P. (2017). The Complete Beginner's Guide to Strength Training. https://www.verywell.com/complete-beginners-guide-to-strength-training-1229585

www.ingramcontent.com/pod-product-compliance
Lightning Source LLC
Chambersburg PA
CBHW061745270326
41928CB00011B/2375